P9-DWB-726

CALGARY PUBLIC LIBRARY

SEP —   2010

"The HIV/AIDS pandemic doesn't just affect millions; it affects them one at a time. Shane's story will stay in your mind and more in your heart."

—John Ortberg, author and pastor,
Menlo Park Presbyterian Church

"If ever there was a page-turning human story, this is one. But Shane Stanford has written less his story than God's story— a story of grace, mercy, and faithfulness as convicting as it is captivating."

—Leonard Sweet, Drew Theological School,
George Fox University, *Sermons.com*

"I'm always on the lookout for stories about the church living up to her identity and calling. This is a story about an individual, a family, a disease—but it's also a story about the church: she stumbles at points, fails in moments, and then ultimately does the hard, good work of opening her doors to a disease against which her doors have been long closed. By the end of the story, I was proud of the church and thankful for Shane and his family's gentle persistence, pushing the church in exactly the right direction."

—Shauna Niequist, author of *Cold Tangerines*

"Shane Stanford joins an impressive line of Mississippi writers who know how to tell a story, including their own. And what a story he tells. There is intrigue, love, fear, disappointment, forgiveness, and setback. But it is primarily a story of grace—God's unfathomable grace and the human grace it inspires. This is a story well worth telling—told very well."

—Lovett H. Weems Jr., Distinguished Professor of Church
Leadership, Wesley Theological Seminary

A POSITIVE LIFE

A POSITIVE LIFE

Living with HIV
as a Pastor, Husband, and Father

Shane Stanford

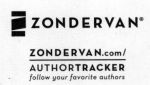

ZONDERVAN.com/
AUTHORTRACKER
follow your favorite authors

ZONDERVAN

A Positive Life
Copyright © 2010 by Shane Stanford

This title is also available as a Zondervan ebook.
Visit www.zondervan.com/ebooks.

This title is also available in a Zondervan audio edition.
Visit www.zondervan.fm.

Requests for information should be addressed to:

Zondervan, *Grand Rapids, Michigan 49530*

Library of Congress Cataloging-in-Publication Data

Stanford, Shane, 1970 –
    A positive life : living with HIV as a pastor, husband, and father / Shane
Stanford.
       p. cm.
    ISBN 978-0-310-29292-0 (jacketed)
    ISBN 978-0-203-85155-5 (ebk)
    1. AIDS (Disease) — Patients — Religious life. 2. AIDS (Disease) — Religious
aspects — Christianity. 3. Stanford, Shane, 1970 – 4. AIDS
(Disease) — Patients — United States — Biography. I. Title.
BV4910.3.S73   2010
248.8'61969792 — dc22
                                       2009046397

All Scripture quotations unless otherwise indicated are taken from the *New Revised
Standard Version* of the Bible, copyright ©1989, Division of Christian Education of the
National Council of the Churches of Christ in the United States of America, and are used
by permission. All rights reserved.

Any Internet addresses (websites, blogs, etc.) and telephone numbers printed in this
book are offered as a resource. They are not intended in any way to be or imply an
endorsement by Zondervan, nor does Zondervan vouch for the content of these sites
and numbers for the life of this book.

All rights reserved. No part of this publication may be reproduced, stored in a retrieval
system, or transmitted in any form or by any means — electronic, mechanical, photocopy,
recording, or any other — except for brief quotations in printed reviews, without the prior
permission of the publisher.

Cover photography: Getty Images® / Robin Bartholick
Interior design: Michelle Espinoza

Printed in the United States of America

10 11 12 13 14 15 16 • 22 21 20 19 18 17 16 15 14 13 12 11 10 9 8 7 6 5 4 3 2 1

For those who make life matter —
strong,
steady,
enthusiastic.
Every day is useful.
Thank you.

And
for Pokey —
No ordinary fairytale
for an extraordinary life.
I love you.

CONTENTS

Foreword by Kay Warren   11

More Than the Sum of What We Can Say   15

1. The Day Before   29

2. Somewhere This Side of Normal   47

3. The Shallow Water   57

4. T Cells and Thresholds   75

5. Putting Our Future Where Our Faith Is   87

6. Conversations for Other Places   103

7. The Cost of What We Cannot Afford   123

8. Glimpses of a Straight Line So Precious   139

9. A Matter of the Heart   161

10. The First Day of the Rest of My Life   175

11. What Happens Next, Daddy?   183

Afterword by Pokey Stanford   191

Speech at the Global AIDS Summit   197

Nine Lessons from a Positive Life:
A Study and Reflection Guide   201

Acknowledgments   215

For Further Reading   217

FOREWORD

My journey into HIV/AIDS advocacy began inauspiciously one spring day in 2002 when I picked up a newsmagazine and read a heartbreaking story of how HIV/AIDS was viciously tearing apart families all over Africa. Up until that moment in time, I had not paid much attention to the greatest humanitarian crisis our world has ever seen. I'm not proud of my attitude; in fact, I still grieve today over the years I wasted in ignorance and apathy. When God finally got my attention with the terrible suffering of those living with HIV and AIDS, he broke my heart into a million pieces. I realized that they mattered to God, and if they mattered to him, they must matter to me. I can no longer live my life unaware or uninvolved with the 33 million men, women, and children who bear the burden of being HIV positive.

Because of my commitment to doing what I can to help the church of Jesus Christ be on the front lines of prevention, treatment, care, and support of people living with HIV and AIDS, I am always on the lookout for others who share those same values. On one of our family vacations, my husband brought a stack of books to read, including Shane Stanford's *The Seven Next Words of Christ*. The title caught my eye, and I thought it would be a pleasant way to spend a few hours. As I glanced at the back cover, I was thrilled to discover that Shane was an HIV positive pastor in Mississippi (The strangest things get me excited these days!). I couldn't wait to get home to contact Shane and learn more about him.

After Shane and I emailed a few times, I was certain that he was supposed to come and give his testimony at the 2006 Global Summit on AIDS and the Church. For three years in a row, Saddleback Church hosted the Global Summit as an opportunity for those who were just learning about HIV ministry to increase their knowledge, for those who were veterans of HIV ministry to share their expertise, and for all to connect with others in fighting the good fight. I loved Shane's pastor's heart, his passion for God, and his articulate way of bringing truth to every conversation.

Sure enough, Shane moved the hearts of those attending the Global Summit — not just his fellow pastors or others who were HIV positive. His voice was strong, full of confidence in the God he trusts. He didn't sugarcoat what it's like to live with HIV. He presented the reality of the struggle with a virus that is constantly seeking a way to destroy him and of the pain that comes from the uncertainty of fragile health. When he finished, the crowd roared their appreciation, for he inspired them to live their lives with hope.

Like his speech at the Global Summit, *A Positive Life* is a real message from a real man. Shane warmly invites the reader into his intense physical journey with hemophilia, HIV, and hepatitis C, as well as into his very intimate marriage journey with his wife, Pokey. Again, no sugarcoating the reality of marriage problems, failure, and sin. But at the end of the day, Shane's story is not so much about pain, suffering, loss, and grief as it is about perseverance, faith, hope, and love.

I'm grateful that God has allowed my path to cross with Shane's; I consider him a friend and a brother, a fellow bond slave of Jesus Christ. My prayer is that you will draw strength, courage, and hope for your life journey from Shane's story. I have.

Kay Warren
Founder, HIV/AIDS Initiative
Saddleback Church
Lake Forest, California

Introduction

MORE THAN THE SUM OF WHAT WE CAN SAY

The positive life is more mosaic than a measurable frame of goods and bads, joys and sorrows, laughter and tears. It is discovered through the composition of its diversity—no single color or component can adequately define a mosaic or its image anymore than one hardship or achievement can or should define life or its nature. And thus, it is these diverse colors, circumstances, victories, and struggles, glimpses brought together—more than simply a snapshot of one image, success or failure—that unveil this life. We are more than the sum of what we can visualize ... describe ... accomplish ... or even endure.

—Journal entry, December 6, 2006

My grandfather didn't talk much, but when he did, his words were wise and strong. People said they'd seen him cry only twice: when his mother died and when he first held his grandson. Tears were difficult for my grandfather. He preferred to live life with logic and decorum. But sometimes life doesn't work that way. And when it didn't, my grandfather taught me how to live when life becomes uncertain.

I spent a lot of time at my grandfather's table, week in and week out for the better part of twenty-eight years. Mr. Earl's dining room table was about more than just a good meal; it was an opportunity to glean wisdom from this quiet, faithful man, to catch a glimmer of what God wants us to be.

One of Grandpa's favorite phrases was "If you break it, you own it." My grandfather believed every part of life costs something—good or bad. We invest ourselves in life and many times we do the breaking by our words, actions, or decisions. Sometimes, though, life breaks us, and we spend the better part of our days piecing our lives back together.

Some people don't believe a broken life can mean much. But I have learned that when life breaks us, we can work to own it before it owns us. In the process, we discover what authentic value and self-worth mean in this world and what really matters. These moments don't come cheap, but their value is measureless.

I was six years old when I learned of my parents' divorce. Sitting on the front lawn of the house we rented, I cried at the news that my parents were separating. I had been kept in the dark about our family's problems. I never saw it coming. But if there was a bright spot in my parents' divorce, it was that my relationship with my grandfather deepened. My father was a good man but was focused on his career. When it came time for my biweekly visits with my dad, under the rules of the custody, I found myself staying the entire weekend with my grandparents.

Over the course of those ten years or so, my grandfather and I became very close; my grandfather was my hero, mentor, and best friend. Sunday mornings were especially important. I would wake up and race to my grandparents' bed where I'd crawl in and wait for my grandfather to fix me a "coffee-milk"—a concoction of half coffee and half milk. We watched the news together. My grandparents didn't shield me from the world as much as my parents did. During those Sunday mornings, I confronted such issues as the Iran hostage crisis and the death of John Lennon and caught my first glimpse of Madonna. That is also when I first heard a news report about homosexuals dying of a mysterious immune system disorder.

After coffee and the news, my grandfather cooked pancakes in a large cast-iron skillet. The pancakes covered my entire plate, and I ate every bite. As soon as breakfast was finished, my grandfather and I would get in his red Chevy pickup and head out to the field. Depending on the season, we would pick fresh peaches from the orchard or check on the cows. Sometimes we would just sit together and watch the morning pass. These times belonged to the two of us. Eventually we would head home and get ready for church, but no matter what the preacher said in the sermon that morning, nothing was more spiritual or formational than those times shared outdoors.

Mostly they were quiet times, but as I grew older, I would ask advice about different situations. Although my grandfather did not expound — he hated long-winded responses to anything — he gave solid, straightforward advice, the kind I knew I could trust the moment I heard it. His favorite phrase was "We always have a choice to do the right thing." My grandfather had strong opinions, but he was not closed-minded. He gifted me with room to disagree and to form my own opinions. However, Grandpa always expected that I do the right thing by others and by God. "Sport, we always have a choice," he would say. And then, as though I needed extra emphasis, he would look me in the eyes and repeat, "Always!"

I was less than a year old when doctors discovered I had hemophilia. My family realized that this would not only affect my ability to clot and heal, but my life as well. My family loved sports and was always active outdoors; having a child who was a hemophiliac would certainly affect their lifestyle. They spent a great deal of time making life as normal as possible for me, and my grandfather in particular went out of his way to find safe sports that we could do together. That's how we discovered golfing.

When my grandfather realized that golf offered me the ability to compete without the danger of contact and getting hurt, he bought me my first set of clubs, taught me the rules, and made a point of playing with me every chance he could. Over the years, golf, like our Sunday mornings, became sacred; when the fields and orchards became too much for Grandpa to tend, we would hold our "special Sunday meetings" on a scenic hill overlooking a local golf course.

The meetings were not usually profound, but there were the occasional "aha" moments when I would see an issue a different way and change my mind because of what my grandfather said. During one particular summer, emotions between my parents became strained. My mother, along with my stepfather, was upset with my father over child support payment issues. My father was equally upset over visitation rights. Stuck in the middle, of course, was me. I understood early that whether my parents intended it, I was the pawn in the game. And many times, I played the role of the emotional tool maneuvered to see which one would achieve checkmate.

Though my grandfather was naturally predisposed to favor the issues of his son, he never spoke a negative or harsh word to me about my mother or my stepfather. I was the primary issue for my grandfather, and so when we would talk on those Sunday mornings, it was about how I was seeing the world. My grandfather was the one person in my life who I knew was listening to my concerns.

Several weeks after I was diagnosed with HIV, my family told my grandfather the news. He left the room immediately after being told. The news devastated him. In the late 1980s, AIDS was a death sentence. Although experts feverishly hoped for new drugs, people were dying at an alarming rate, and the future did not seem hopeful.

In the weeks following the news, I struggled to get used to the diagnosis. At first, I avoided any discussion of the disease and tried to resume a normal routine. I was in the middle of my junior golf season and had qualified to play on the local university's junior golf team. But it was hard to practice, hitting golf balls over and over again, knowing that deep inside this virus was waiting to kill me. Not much could be done. Everyone knew that HIV (which was a fairly new way of discussing AIDS, since the test was so new) was a death sentence. There were no medicines other than a few drugs used for fighting the symptoms of the opportunistic infections. Other than that, HIV/AIDS meant dying.

I had always dealt with my hemophilia and with injuries very well. I was strong and stoic. It was easy to talk about faith in God and to "be an example" when you knew deep down that the disease wasn't going to kill you. I remember thinking what a fraud I felt like, proclaiming this great faith of how God could handle any situation—until this one. Now I was struggling. I couldn't pray or read my Bible, and my heart felt very distant from God. I had always been able to talk to him as if he were standing next to me. Now God felt very far away.

I remember wondering how others in my family were taking the news. My mother was strong, but I could hear her cry late at night. My father didn't talk much about it, only offering an "It's going to be okay" from time to time. My stepfather, who by that time had become like my own father, kept the routine going and comforted my mother. They were dealing with the same feelings I felt, except they weren't the patient. But now that I have children, I think that must have been even worse.

One night while reluctantly reading my Bible—which I did a great deal during that time, because no matter my feelings, I had been taught it was the thing to do—I read through the passage about Jesus in the garden of Gethsemane, when he begged the Father to take the cup of suffering away from him.

The agony was palpable, and anyone who reads the passage feels for Jesus during this scene. But as I thought especially about my mom, I felt for the Father too. Here was his Son asking him to help, but the Father knew that, given the circumstances, the die was cast and there was nothing to do. I wonder what heaven was like at that moment.

Anyway, we all traipsed around doing our normal things and trying to make sense of the situation, but there was little sense to be made. The news was devastating. I had overcome numerous obstacles in my life and had kept a positive attitude. Now a positive diagnosis threatened not only my body, but also how I saw the world and especially how I saw God.

But when people with personalities like mine (cholerics, type As, fires, etc.) are faced with dismal situations, we try to find the center of the story and the best place to land. I tried to resume a sense of normalcy, but all too often I woke up at night gripped by the realization of what my diagnosis meant. It was almost more than a teenage boy could endure. Just days before, I had gone to bed as the captain of the golf team and president of my class, knowing that I was dating the prettiest girl in school. I had dreams of law school and a life in politics. Now I was dying at the hands of what could only be considered as the leprosy of our time. No matter who was around, it was a very lonely time.

The first weekend I spent with my grandparents after the diagnosis was awkward. My disease was not discussed. No one wanted to be the first to mention the diagnosis. After Sunday breakfast, my grandfather asked me to take a ride with him. We drove the familiar road to the hill overlooking the golf course and sat together in silence.

My grandfather's habit when we would arrive was to say an

"open-eye" prayer. He liked to say that no one else would want him to say an open-eye prayer, because prayer was supposed to be with our eyes closed and our heads bowed. But sitting here or in the orchard, my grandfather would ask, "How can we pray to God and be thankful for all we have and see and be afraid to look up and actually take it all in?"

My grandfather's reasoning always made sense to me when we were sitting there, though I dared not try the open-eye prayer anywhere else. Looking up also meant making our prayers more about God than about ourselves, which so many prayers seemed to be. So we would pray, looking up, around, and at each other. It was always a great moment, filled with laughter, smiles, and an occasional loving stare from a grandfather to his grandson.

On this particular day, my grandfather finished the prayer and then took my hand. He had looked over at me several times. We knew there was more in the air than just the breeze and much more to discuss.

Finally, my grandfather broke the silence: "What are you going to do with this thing?" He never used the letters *HIV* or the word *AIDS*, and he never talked about sickness or disease. But I knew exactly what he was talking about.

"I don't know. There's no cure," I said, looking down while messing with a blade of grass. "There is not much of a choice."

"You always have a choice," my grandfather said, his voice steady. He was straightforward in his words but not gruff or difficult in his tone. He just wanted me to hear and pay attention.

"What choice do I have?" I asked. There didn't seem to be many choices on my end. In fact, the doctors had not given any, and most, if not everyone in my life, were walking around as though resigned to the fact that there were no choices available.

"Sometimes," I finally added, "I feel like running as fast as I can. I am not sure where I would go, but just to see if I could outrun this feeling of loneliness and dread in my life." My grandfather was listening.

"And then there are times when I just want to lie down and let it be over. Some days it is hard to find a reason to feel joyful again. That scares me more than the disease."

My grandfather had looked back at the horizon. I could tell he was thinking.

"I know there is a lot to consider over the next weeks. Dr. Kent is telling me a lot about what I need to think about in terms of my treatment. So I am trying to get the right info and make good decisions. But choices?" I asked. "About life ... really, about life? I don't know about that."

My grandfather and I sat there for a few moments. I was trying to be honest with him about where my heart was in this news and in this whole fight. I had gone through a lot in my life, but this was different. The face of this disease was bigger than all of us put together. And the impact was not just about my life, but about so many others in my family. Remember, this was all being done in secret, since most people could not at that point in the disease's timeline get their brains around the idea of what my being HIV positive would mean for them, our family, and our community.

My grandfather shifted to turn more toward me. He leaned against the ground with his left arm so that he could look me in the eye. "If anybody has a right to get in the corner and have a pity party about this, it's you. It's a very raw deal, and I can't tell you that I understand it or have even begun to confront my anger over it. But as bad as this seems—and I know it's bad—you have a choice to make. You can get in that corner, and if you want me to, I will get in there with you." My grandfather paused. I had never heard him talk about giving up or giving in to anything. But here he was with tears in his eyes, saying that he would crawl into that pity party hole with me if that is where I went and he needed to go.

"But I know you, maybe better than anyone. I know what is in your heart and deep in your soul, and I think you are going to make a choice other than pity, retreat, or surrender. I think you are going to live each day to the fullest with everything you have. I think you are going to take each day, no matter how many you have, and make something of it. No one can ask any more of you."

He stopped and looked into my eyes. "And son, I think your making *that* choice will mean something someday."

A DIFFERENT STAGE

Nearly twenty years after that moment with my grandfather, I was asked to share my story for a few minutes at the Saddleback Global AIDS Summit, founded by Kay and Rick Warren. By this time in my ministry, I had shared my story hundreds of times. My grandfather had been right. The story itself made a difference for people, even when it was not particularly welcome and when people did not know what to do with it. And I had developed a good reputation as a speaker who loved to move while he talked, share from his heart, and talk about this story with a certain animation that kept people involved. After all, in my mind, the goal was for my story to prick something in their own story that would cause them to see the unfailing love of

God in their journey and then move them to action. And I had told the story so many times that it was more than just a speech; it had become part of my natural movement when I talked. Thus, I rarely spoke with anything other than a few brief notes, a microphone, and two unleashed, moving hands. The Saddleback people, however, were squeezing a lot of info and speakers into a very compressed time frame. I was scheduled to speak in the first session in between remarks by Rick and Kay. So I wrote my remarks down word for word. I wanted this speech to be less about my delivery and more about the meaning of the story. This speech was personal.

What developed was four minutes about how HIV/AIDS had dominated my life, shaped my worldview, informed my faith, and redesigned my view of others. I was making sense of my story and the lessons it has taught me. My illness is not a part of me; rather, it *is* me in so many positive ways — my marriage, my family, my vocation, my faith. HIV/AIDS has taught me simple things about living, about how to love more and better, and about how to serve beyond my own interests. It has carved away my prejudices and fears and shaped my view of God and God's people — the latter, unfortunately, often in a negative light. HIV/AIDS is my common story and my moral voice — the deepest place where God worked his presence in me.

From the doctor's room where, as a sixteen-year-old kid, I learned my HIV status, to the conference room of the church that would not accept me as their pastor; and from the grieving rooms where I said good-bye to friends, to the hospital rooms where my wife buried her head in my chest and cried, HIV/AIDS has been my means of grace more than my wound of sorrow.

I feel more familiar than angry. As much as the disease has pushed and torn at me, I know myself, the world, and God's heart better. I would prefer to be healthy and disease-free, but I have become content with the struggle—maybe even, at times, not wishing to trade it away. Illness has refined my soul; and life, people, and goals mean different things because of its presence.

As Rick finished his opening remarks, I remember my heart was about to pound out of my chest. I walked to the podium. Rick hugged me and said, "Thanks for being here. You are a blessing." But the real blessing was being anywhere, anytime at all. I couldn't help but think that my grandfather would like this moment. And I couldn't help but remember those who along the way had meant so much and, for one reason or another, could not be there. This had not just been my fight or my battle. I looked to my right and saw my wife, Pokey, sitting in the audience. She smiled a huge smile, and I saw her wink at me. And looking forward, I saw the media, cameras, and over two thousand Summit participants who had their own stories and war wounds.

Standing at that podium in front of the world, I realized that, like so many others in that room, I had met the enemy over many years, and I had been fortunate enough to prosper. Yes, the disease attacked my body, but because of the disease, I attacked life with an understanding of the brokenness through which we, like Paul, can declare God's grace to be sufficient. No, it wasn't easy. There are still times I want to take off running or lie down and give up. Did all go as planned? I am afraid not. But the story showed that we had at least made the choice for something better and had, to our best, lived it faithfully, even when we would get it horribly wrong. Regardless, the story is real, and it is mine.

LIVING POSITIVE

I have lived now nearly a quarter of a century "positive." That is the lingo we attach to someone who is HIV positive, whether we say it from within the HIV community or from the sidelines. It means many things to many different people. It is a test result, a way of life, a question of morality, a lifestyle, a badge, a condition, or a burden.

For me it has been all of those things at one time. However, "positive" is, more than anything, the story of my life. The lessons of my story are about the people who made—and still make—my life worth living. A common thread binds us together: the broken, forgotten, rediscovered, and redeemed present within us all. *Their story*, *your story*, *my story*, and *God's story* become *our story*. Recognizing this bond is what defines a life well lived, regardless of the details. For some of us, the facts and figures are daunting and difficult; for others, life has been mostly comfortable and without much struggle. But the story remains, and how we assimilate it, analyze it, calibrate it, and share it determines in so many ways and places how we will live it and how others will learn by it.

In the following pages, you will hear a lot about my story, about the things I celebrate and the things I regret. You will learn secrets from my past but also discover hopeful places where the secrets and regret did not win. You will also meet a lot of people who kept me alive because they made life so important and wonderful for me. And of course, you will see Jesus and how much I love him and how much, in spite of so much I have not gotten right, I believe he loves me. At times this story will encourage you, and at other times it will push you away, because I want better for you and for those I love. But more than anything, it will speak honestly about life — my life, your life, and God's life. By the end, I hope the authenticity will have touched you and you will, if nothing else, know that I meant what I wrote and that it matters to me. And I believe you will see that my life is positive for more than my diagnosis or for even how I live with the illness. I think you will see that it is positive because when I decided to show up, I found that God was already there. Likewise, when you are meandering through your own maze of life, look up — God is there with you too.

At the end of the book, I share lessons born from the earlier pages that might be helpful as you navigate your own story. These lessons will sometimes be easily relatable to your journey yet at other times seem quite foreign.

Thank you for reading my story. I trust it will help you see your own story — and our story with God — a bit more clearly, and that you will see the positive elements in your own life and the places you should celebrate and remember. And I hope that you will see that we always have a choice to see the world differently, to see people differently, and to make a better way. We don't have to live, much as we generally pray, with our eyes closed and our heads looking down, hoping that the next blow won't hurt so much. No, God wants us to look up, see the crowd, take in the scenery, and in spite of every voice or inkling that says it isn't possible, make another choice.

So, enjoy. I look forward to reading your own version — of your story, God's story, our story — one day.

Chapter 1

THE DAY BEFORE

Dear God, Ms. Gandy, my Sunday school teacher, said you said we could ask for anything and that you would listen. I mostly talk to you by praying, but this is important, so I thought I would write it down....

—First journal entry, January 19, 1979

Trauma changes us. I watched a woman on the news describe the year since she had survived a plane crash in Chicago. She said the event had profoundly changed the way she viewed her world; she spent more time with her family and tried to enjoy the "every-dayness" of things. Her relationships, language, and worldview were framed in the context of before the accident and after it.

"You can't make sense of the whole of your life unless you understand the magnitude of how much changes when the world turns upside down," she said. "You may not remember all of the details or circumstances, but you most certainly know the timeline."

When we try to understand *today*, it matters what happened *before*.

THE DAYS BEFORE

Growing up a hemophiliac, I spent a great deal of time in the hospital. Thankfully, my diagnosis was mild by other comparisons, and I only needed medical attention when I was hurt or having a procedure. As most little boys do, I often did things that were either unwise or downright stupid. Although my parents kept me from playing most organized contact sports, I played a lot of backyard football, baseball, basketball, and soccer. Thus, I was always hurt from some shot or lick I took, and I found myself in the emergency room much more often than my mother liked.

The nurses and doctors at the local emergency room were more than just my caretakers when it came time for Factor VIII (the medicine used to treat the hemophilia); they were my family. Whenever I got hurt, they would stitch me up, give me a dose of Factor, and send me on my way. Because Factor was so expensive and had to be administered through an IV, local emergency rooms became the places for most hemophiliacs to receive their doses, especially the mild ones like me.

Though I was mild, I saw the nurses on a regular basis. I was always doing something that hemophiliacs (or most children) in general shouldn't do. Once I tried to ramp a parked car on my mountain bike. I made it — halfway. The other half was me rolling off the side of the car and hitting the ground. I also enjoyed building forts, that would, for one reason or another, lead to a nail stuck in my hand or a bruised knee from the rope swing. And I enjoyed sports of any kind. Though I tried to be as careful as possible, I wanted to be as normal as everyone else, which meant taking an elbow to the chin in basketball or a bruised rib in football or tearing ligaments in my ankle chasing a fly ball in baseball. Yes, the nurses saw me on a regular basis, and I took my fair share of scolding and lectures from them about how I should be careful and use "what little of my mind I apparently had" they would say. But I think deep down they liked seeing me. I was always hurt, of course, but I was just a normal boy.

It was during one of those visits that I met a new pediatrician named Dr. Ronnie Kent, an extremely upbeat man whose sense of humor and kindness made any patient feel better. I was in the ER from a water slide accident — rushing water plus concrete plus a three-hundred-pound man racing behind me. My forehead caught the brunt of the landing, and I received a "goose egg" the size of a fifty-cent piece, which immediately swelled and turned purple.

My stepfather arrived at the hospital just after I was taken for a CAT scan. He was told to go to the basement of the hospital to find me. Radiology and the morgue were located on the same floor. As the elevator opened, my stepfather saw the sign — MORGUE — and thought I had died. He stood there, frozen, wondering how he would tell my mother.

Eventually someone directed him to the CAT scan lab around the corner. The doctors kept me at the hospital for a few days, and all the while my mother was on bed rest at home after delivering my sister, Whitney. It was a stressful time, but when Dr. Kent walked into the room, I immediately felt at ease. From the beginning, Ronnie and I had an instant rapport. He was a devout Christian who talked openly about his faith, and he spent a lot of time talking to me and my family. Given the complexities of my health, this meant a great deal to us. Dr. Kent became my friend as well as my doctor.

It was during the course of my all-too-regular childhood visits to Dr. Kent that he first mentioned AIDS. The nation was becoming aware of the disease that was affecting primarily gay men in large cities. There were concerns that the disease had found its way to the blood supply, particularly to the hemophiliac community through our medicines, all of which are made from human blood products. Dr. Kent reassured my parents he believed everything would be fine, but just in case, he recommended we try to avoid Factor as much as possible. He suggested using several alternatives, including older remedies for hemophilia not made of human blood, as well as hormone drugs that were known to raise clotting factors. Given the lack of any formal test for AIDS antibodies and the long-term development of the disease once a person has seroconverted (become positive with the disease), many of us thought we had bypassed any real issue concerning infection or contamination. So, as with most issues not acutely impacting our lives, I mostly forgot about the implications. I was told to be *careful*. That was no small feat for an adolescent boy, but I tried.

Over the next couple of years, I *was* careful, surprisingly so. There were a few injuries here and there, but nothing that would require significant use of Factor. My health remained strong. The new medicines for raising clotting levels worked well, giving hope that my Factor intake would be minimal until a safe supply could be developed.

Life was as normal as any hemophiliac could enjoy. I heard stories of hemophiliacs whose lives were otherwise, hemophiliacs like young Ryan White who contracted AIDS and was kicked out of his school in Indiana. I rooted for him each step of the way, even as I was secretly relieved that I didn't have to go through what he endured—and grateful I had been spared infection.

There were other stories too. The saga of the Ray family in Florida was most disconcerting, because their house was burned after a series of death threats. *All because they have a disease?* I asked my mother. I could tell that she was horrified by the news of what others were doing to these families. We would pray for them, but again, we remained thankful that we had somehow missed the force of this storm.

Just prior to the seventh grade, I was diagnosed with keritikonis, a hereditary and degenerative malformation of the corneas. Whereas most people's corneas are round, mine were pointed and caused significant vision problems. Over time, corrective lenses were of no use and the only alternative was a corneal transplant. Without it, my vision would deteriorate until I was legally blind.

Until then, no one in Mississippi had performed a corneal transplant on a hemophiliac. Although corneal surgeries do not experience a lot of bleeding and healing happens at a faster rate than in most other areas of the body, there was a laundry list of concerns for transplants on a hemophiliac. Several doctors refused to take the case. The one who finally agreed was a brilliant, fearless physician in Jackson, Mississippi. Her reputation was impeccable, and she had a penchant for taking difficult cases. She performed my surgery on Halloween 1986. The procedure went well, and almost immediately I regained some sight in my eye. I awoke from surgery thrilled to be seeing again and thankful that complications from the hemophilia were minimal.

However, two months later, I returned because of problems with stitches. The surgery had to be repeated. This was a setback, especially to my spirits. The vision in my other eye had deteriorated by this time, so I was literally blind in one eye and couldn't see out of the other. It was a difficult time emotionally. The prior spring I had finished second in the state high school golf championships, and there was talk of college golf scholarships. Now, months later, I could scarcely navigate my daily routines, much less hit a golf ball.

Even then I saw glimpses of God at work in my life. My hematologist was Indian and even smaller and feistier than my eye surgeon. She was very direct. Concerned that I was spending too much time moping in my hospital room, she insisted that I take a stroll around the ward. Despite my protests, I was sternly booted out of bed by this four-feet-eleven-inch drill sergeant in a doctor's coat.

On one of my forced strolls, I met Kathryn. Through an open door, I saw her sitting on the edge of her bed. Kathryn's eyes radiated an unbelievable blue, but they were no match for her smile. She spoke with crisp words punctuated by a dry, subtle laugh that made me laugh with her. The pediatric ward at the university hospital was filled with sad cases and mostly younger children. The circular building was old, and there were few modern conveniences other than a television in each room. Add to this the fact that I couldn't see very well and that I had few visitors (the hospital was eighty miles from my hometown), and I was craving interaction with anyone remotely my age and with any sense of conversation ability. Kathryn was a welcome sight, for she could talk on any number of topics, from politics and religion (my favorites) to Southeastern conference football. We were both sixteen, and I was intrigued and intimidated by this self-confident young woman. She was the kind of girl I either wanted to marry or elect president. Or both.

After Kathryn's eyes and her smile, the next thing I noticed was the bandage around her head. Kathryn suffered from an inoperable brain tumor. While other sixteen-year-old girls were worrying about what clothes to wear or who to date, Kathryn spent her days dealing with treatments, though I was never fully aware of exactly what, and resting. All I knew was that she spent most of her mornings down in the radiology department and would come back exhausted. She rested most of the afternoons and by early evening felt well enough to talk. The routine of treatments, meds, and doctor visits were visibly taxing and difficult. And often Kathryn felt sick from the side effects. Yet her perspective on life was wide and generous. From the moment I met her, I was amazed by her ability to look beyond the difficul-ties of her illness and maintain hope.

Although the doctors assured Kathryn's family there was nothing they could do to save her life, she continued to fight the odds. She was a nurses' favorite, partly because of her attitude but also because, along with yours truly, she was the oldest child on the floor.

In addition to hope, faith was one of Kathryn's most notice-able attributes. She spoke of God in such personal terms that even the most ardent atheist would feel a connection to God or at least want to know more. Kathryn's faith wasn't a crutch, but a part of life as necessary as breath. My self-pity quickly gave way to awe as this fellow sojourner prayed for, encouraged, and consoled me. Her unshakable optimism never failed to stun me. I remember then, as now, wanting to achieve that kind of hope and faith in my own life. Once when I stopped at Kathryn's room, I found her reading *Mere Christianity* by C. S. Lewis. She read me the section about humanity not being able to identify a crooked line unless we could conceive of a straight line. When she finished, she proceeded to talk about evil and good and about how so many of the things we see in this world naturally fit into one category or the other. Years later, as a pastor, I wouldn't think such a discussion so dramatic, but for two sixteen-year-old kids, it was remarkable. Kathryn loaned me her book, and it sits on my bookshelf to this day.

Why would a sixteen-year-old girl be reading the theological works of C. S. Lewis or, as I would later discover, Bonhoeffer or Augustine? Part of it was that Kathryn was just that bright and inquisitive. But part of it was because of what the world had thrown at her. She was not on an ordinary journey, and the issues she faced couldn't be neatly packaged into rights and wrongs, goods and bads. Kathryn, more than anyone, understood that most of life's conversations take place in the middle, in the gray, in the nuance. I would appreciate this much more months later when I received my diagnosis, knowing from the years and miles since that life is much more than the sum of the words we can say.

Near the end of my hospital stay, the cries from Kathryn's room reached a frightening pitch as her seizures worsened. Her pain must have been unbelievable. However, by the next day, Kathryn, although weakened, displayed the same grace and peace as before. It is still hard to describe the courage and valor she showed. I would arrive at her room to find her sitting in bed with the same smile as so many days before. Sometimes her voice was weaker or her face more drawn from the strain and weariness, but never her spirit and never her sense of faith and presence. She would always invite me in, and we would spend the next few hours talking.

Our last conversation took place shortly after a church youth group visited our hospital ward. Expecting to find only small children, the group members, many of them our own age, dressed in Halloween costumes to hand out candy and other treats to sick children. Kathryn and I caused quite a stir as the visiting youth barged through our doors, only to find two of their peers sitting, somewhat overgrown, in our beds. The looks on their faces ranged between shock and the look you see when a performer knows the show has gone awry but barrels through anyway. These kids had been sent to minister to the "children" of the pediatric ward, never expecting to find their peers. But I remember every one of them regaining their composure long enough to try to cheer us up. Kathryn commented on the hilarious looks on their faces but also the obvious kindness in their hearts. At that point, I realized that I had never seen any young person other than me and these kids in Kathryn's room. Over the course of my stay, my best friends had visited, but I had not seen anyone for Kathryn. I asked her father about this later (a bold act for me at that age), and he said that Kathryn had been sick for so long that many of her friends had gotten back into the routines of their own lives, and that apart from a few kids in her youth group, most of Kathryn's real acquaintances were adults, until, of course, I showed up.

The day I left the hospital, I made one last visit to Kathryn's room. I told her I would take good care of her C. S. Lewis book and that we needed to stay in touch. She said I would soon get back into my routine and forget all about her. "But that is what should happen," she said. "Life goes on like that." Of course, I protested, and I really meant it. I wanted to stay in touch. Kathryn impacted my life, not just in those days, but I would learn later how much.

I arrived home to friends and neighbors checking on me and to the rush of the holiday season. I sent a couple of letters to Kathryn over the Thanksgiving holiday but did not get a return. I even tried calling the number she had given me but was told by who I believe was an aunt that Kathryn had gone on vacation with her family. "Was she doing well?" I asked the woman. "As well as could be expected," she replied. I didn't ask what she meant. I wish I had, because when I returned to the hospital two months later for another eye surgery, no one could tell me about her. I had not heard about Kathryn. It was as though she had vanished.

The whole situation was so strange. For someone whose story

had changed my perspective during that difficult time to simply fall out of my life seemed so odd. Her example and life had been what impacted me most. How could someone with such trials and difficulties as hers possess such a beautiful perspective on the world? I couldn't answer those questions at that point in my life, but I believe God sent Kathryn to help me start not only asking them but also pondering their impact. Life is about questions, these kind and so many others. Kathryn helped me see that even with so much going wrong, we are given the choice of perspective, a sentiment my grandfather would echo months later. Kathryn was my angel, sent from God to prick my soul to start wrestling, even though I had no idea what with or when it would all matter.

But the questions and example that Kathryn was modeling for me and introducing me to were in response to other scenarios happening in my life that I did not know about at the time. And looking back, it is these two life-changing segments of events and relationships—one with a brave, sixteen-year-old girl and the other with doctors and blood tests—that show me how far out in front of us God goes. Nothing comes as a surprise to God. Nothing.

While I was visiting with Kathryn and entranced by her example and life, the daily routines of doctor visits, tests, and rehab provided more than enough for me to worry about. Rest was pretty much elusive in the hospital. There were always doctors in the room asking questions, poking, and prodding, and I endured blood test after blood test—the process became almost routine. As a hemophiliac, I was having my factor levels tested often—white blood counts to test for infections and red blood counts to make sure my iron and platelet levels remained constant. So, with such a variety of blood tests being done, I never would have questioned another test. Doctors reported regularly and were open and honest with us. Factor reports came back at 10:00 a.m. and 4:00 p.m. Later in the evening, the hematologist would check on me, as would the ophthalmologist. These tests and interruptions were all part of my routine.

One day, late in the afternoon, my hematologist stopped by my room and asked my mom, stepfather, and father to step out into the hall. This was unusual; my mom didn't usually hold anything back from me. I was concerned but not particularly worried. My family had built relationships with all of my doctors, and they conversed regularly.

However, when Mom reentered the room, I could tell she had been crying. I asked her what was wrong. My mother hates for people to know she has been crying, usually going to great lengths to pretend that everything is okay. That time, however, she just looked at me without trying to hide what was more than obvious on her face.

"It's just that your blood-clotting levels are lower than I'd like to see them, and we want you to get better," she said. I knew my family was tired too. They had been with me over the past months throughout all of the surgeries and procedures.

"I will, Mom," I promised her. "It is all going to be okay."

She smiled. She knew that I could no more promise that than I could promise that I would have no more accidents. It just didn't happen that way.

Deep down I knew something else was wrong, but I dismissed it as Mom being tired and overly worried. It wasn't until ten months later that I would discover the truth: I had just tested positive for HIV. Of course, I had no idea that it could be something like this. I had always trusted the adults in my life to tell me the truth. From the time I was a little boy, I needed to trust people. It was part of my DNA, but it was also practical. Much of life was spent with someone sticking a needle in me, and remaining still and allowing people to do their work was necessary. I had fought back a couple of times as a child, and the medical personnel had put restraints on me. It was only after I promised not to fight and allow them to get their job done that I learned how, through clenched teeth, to endure the pain and not ask too many questions. I came to the conclusion that if there was anything I needed to know, they would tell me.

At some point, this idea took root in my psyche, and I trusted the adults in my life implicitly. Sure, not being told something as serious as that I was HIV positive is staggering, and knowing that I went nearly a year before someone finally shared the real drama in my life with me is hard. But what would any of us have done? What else could anyone expect of my parents, considering the impact of that news on them — knowing that no treatment was available, knowing that many people would not understand or may even get violent because of it, and knowing that, with my diseased eyes, I was already under a lot of strain? Sure, there is a part of me that wishes they would have trusted me as much as I trusted them. But as the years have passed, I have learned to read the rest of the story and see the other side too. Life is hard and does not always come at us with perfect intentions or plans laid out. We take what we find and deal with it.

I learned later that my mom cried nearly every day after the diagnosis. Having children myself now, I can't imagine how I would have felt. She almost told me several times over the course of months, but it never seemed to be the right time. Finally, life found its patterns again, and with me doing better each day and showing no signs of any disease, the urgency wore off.

And even with so much filling our lives during that time, once I was dismissed from the hospital, my life returned to my kind of normal. My eyes slowly mended and my sight improved. I was relearning how to function in the world and finding a measure of healing. Helping the process was a girl named Pokey. We had known each other for years, but Pokey and I ran in different circles. Then one day, on a trip to a school convention, she literally landed in my lap. With no seats left in the fifteen-passenger van, Pokey, notorious for running late, arrived just before the doors closed. Teachers were barking at her to find a seat, and so she did—in my lap. There she rode for two hours; no teacher protested, and I wasn't about to either! Within two months, I summoned the courage to ask her to the prom, and the rest, as they say, is history.

I'm not exactly a neutral observer, but my wife is nothing short of striking—when she enters a room, people sit up and take notice. But when Pokey and I started dating, I was legally blind in one eye and wore a patch on the other. I first fell in love with Pokey for other qualities, but I was certainly pleased by what my gradually improving eyesight revealed! I was the nerd who spent most of his time studying in the library or working for the "class cause," while Pokey was the cutie who became famous for her ardent love of life and for her slightly mischievous side. On the surface, no two people could have appeared more different.

Pokey was fun and full of life, a stark contrast to my reserved, quiet demeanor. She helped me enjoy life and not take myself so seriously. I, in her words, "grounded her" and made her think

THE DAY BEFORE 43

about her goals and dreams. We were good for one another. I wasn't looking for a girlfriend any more than she was looking for a boyfriend. We had both been through major heartbreaks the year before and decided that dating was not all it was cracked up to be. Besides, what brought us into each other's life were not the usual romantic notions. I liked the way she laughed and giggled. She liked the way my brow furrowed when I was thinking about something serious. We could sit and either talk or be quiet. It may sound strange, but at sixteen neither of us wanted much more than a genuine friend.

And yet there was something special about Pokey that touched deep into my soul. It is hard to explain the broken edges of life with someone who has never experienced them. Pokey didn't need any explanations. I could tell that she had seen her share of heartbreak. Even at such a young age, we shared a mutual understanding of certain wounded and broken places in our lives. In each other we found a willing friend and an understanding spirit. Pokey and I became inseparable, a couple who were also each other's best friend and biggest fan. Moreover, Pokey supported my search for God's place in my life. We didn't understand it then, but God was building a framework for how he would work through both of us later.

During my eye surgery, my relationship with God had run the gamut from deep resentment and anger to acceptance and love. I spent a lot of time talking to God about my condition. My mother and family were and are very devout in their faith, and I had learned from many previous injuries and tough times to trust that God can teach us through our life circumstances. This period was one of the most important times in my life spiritually. I shared my testimony in a Sunday school class and then, later, at a youth event. Before long, my pastor—and Pokey—persuaded me to preach at our annual youth service.

On May 16, 1987, with a patch on my left eye, I preached my first sermon. It was from Philippians 4:4–7, in which Paul writes, "Do not worry about anything, but in everything by prayer and supplication with thanksgiving let your requests be made known to God. And the peace of God, which surpasses all understanding, will guard your hearts and your minds in Christ Jesus" (vv. 6–7).

I had learned this passage was more than words. As a hemophiliac, I knew what it was like to be in great pain and to spend hours lying in bed in agony over an injury that would take much longer than normal to heal. These moments had been my chance to place my pain in God's hands, and I had talked about that many times. Many people don't realize that hemophiliacs experience excruciating pain during an illness; they associate hemophilia with a cut or bleeding on the outside. But the vast majority of a hemophiliac's problems are because of internal injuries. A hemophiliac's joints and muscles bleed out quickly, and the struggle is not just about stopping the bleeding but also about recovering the site and healing the tissue so that it can be usable or strong again. That is why if an injury to, say, a hemophiliac's ankle is not properly healed and rehabbed, the tissue will remain damaged forever and that person will always have problems using that ankle effectively. Injuries, especially to joints and muscles, are very painful, and there is very little that can be done for them. Most physicians give Factor, but it takes time for the bleeding to stop and then for the injury to heal. There is a lot of discomfort, not to mention a lot of still moments, also excruciating to a child hemophiliac. While I was laid up, I couldn't do much but read and watch movies, which is where my love for books and movies came from.

But more than anything, growing up in pain taught me a lot about how much of this world we can't control. A lot of what we face, we have to barrel through or the pain will get the best of us. The latter is simply not an option. Probably one of my most difficult injuries was a back injury when I was just eight. I was swinging on the monkey bars and lost my grip. I not only landed on my back but on a small stick coming up from the ground. The bleed to my back muscles was severe, and the pain was excruciating. For nearly three weeks, during which time my mom would take me every twelve hours for Factor treatments, I laid on the hardwood floor of my house because it was the only place I could find relief. The doctors never gave me pain medicines, and I've never known why. I just spent my time hurting. I remember once that the muscle was so filled with blood from the hemorrhage that I was in agony and wept and begged my mom to make it stop. "Please, please do something, Mommy," I cried. But there was nothing she could do. We simply had to allow time to pass and healing to occur. I do remember, however, my mother lying down on that floor with me every night and sleeping there for those three weeks. She couldn't make the pain go away, but she wouldn't abandon me either.

Through all of those different injuries, I also learned that the body, the spirit, and the soul don't differ much in how they respond to difficulties. Healing does not come at once; we have to be patient and wait. God's healing passes understanding; it gets down on the floor with us and wipes away our tears and holds us, especially when the aches and pains of life seem too much to bear.

I wanted people to hear that in my sermon. I didn't know how many times I would get to preach, and so I remember working hard to ensure that if folks heard nothing else that evening, they would hear about the love and hope of a God who walks with us in our pain. Before the sermon my nerves made me shake like a leaf. I remember lying on the floor of my bedroom all afternoon prior to the evening service, constantly on the edge of throwing up. I had spoken in front of groups before, but there was something more, something bigger about preaching. I would never lose that feeling, even years and thousands of sermons later. This is not uncommon for pastors to say or feel. Those who believe they would have chosen something else to do for a living if preaching had not chosen them always refer to the delicate balance between sharing God's Word and complete utter terror. That is what I felt that evening. I wanted so much to tell everything that God had meant to me and had done for me in my life. But the message for that evening was about hope and peace. Years later, though I now preach for a living, I still would choose something else except that God has chosen me for this.

As difficult as my sixteenth year of life had been, things were on track again in June of 1987. God had answered my prayers about my relationship with him. I had faced some struggles, but my world seemed normal again and my future appeared limitless. My sight was returning, I was playing golf again, I had preached my first sermon, and I had found the girl of my dreams. I couldn't wait to see what came next.

Chapter 2

SOMEWHERE THIS SIDE OF NORMAL

Played great today. I think I shot a 78. Not bad when you consider I played from the tips. Have the day off from work tomorrow. May play again. Going by to visit Dr. Kent. Should be an easy day.

—Journal entry, June 29, 1987

When we were thirteen years old, my best friend, Jason, and I were playing water volleyball at a last day of school party. Jason asked me, "Have you heard about the disease that is killing gay men in California?" This was a pretty big question for a pimple-faced, girl-obsessed boy from south Mississippi. I had not known my friend to be concerned with such topics before, and I was surprised by the question.

We were like every other boy we knew. We wanted to play sports, talk about girls, and cause our fair share of trouble. The fact that one of us had a disease like hemophilia was never much of an issue unless I was hurt or unless we needed a good excuse to get ourselves out of a jam—which we quite often did. Come to think of it, Jason used my issue of hemophilia for us much more than I did.

"Yes, I have heard about it," I replied. "Why would you ask about that?"

"My mother says that the same disease that is killing those gay men is now making hemophiliacs sick," he said.

"She says that people think the disease may be in the blood supply and that your medicine might have some in it. You haven't felt weird or anything, have you?" This was sixth-grade-boy speak for "Are you okay?"

Your medicine, I thought. No, I had not heard and had never considered that the disease, AIDS, causing such damage in the homosexual community, would find its way to me.

"Our doctors haven't mentioned anything," I said, serving the volleyball.

We didn't discuss the topic again that day or any day for many years, when, by that time, the conversation and the context were much different.

TOO CLOSE TO HOME

The look on Dr. Kent's face said it all. He was nervous and sad but working hard to be neither. He wanted to convey the information but not cause a panic. He wanted to be sensitive but not become overly emotional. He wanted to be a doctor but also a friend. He told me later that this was one of the worst moments of his life.

"Shane, you tested positive for HIV."

I wondered if I had heard him right.

"Are you okay?" he asked.

I didn't know how to answer him. I stood there, almost as if I were outside of myself trying to catch a glimpse of my reaction. At the same time, his expression — part pain, part inquiry — showed me that this was not a dream, though it felt like a nightmare.

"You mean the virus that causes AIDS?" I clarified.

"Yes," he said. "The doctors tested you last October when you had eye surgery, but everyone felt, with all that had been going on, that it was best to wait and let you heal before we told you."

"What does this mean?"

"It means you have the virus that causes AIDS," Dr. Kent replied.

"No, what does that *mean*?" I asked more slowly, trying to wrap my sixteen-year-old brain around this news.

The situation was awkward and uncomfortable. I spoke slowly; so did Dr. Kent. And it was hard for him to make eye contact at first, a rarity for him. This disease did more than infect a person's body; it seeped into the senses. The mere mention of the term sent people reeling. Dr. Kent wasn't pushing back because of the disease but because talking about it sent unmistakable messages about life and death — mostly death.

"Your immune system will get very weak, and there's no treatment for this yet."

"Am I going to die?"

"Shane, we don't want to focus on that...," Dr. Kent started.

"Dr. Kent," I interjected, "am I going to die from this?"

"Probably," he said quietly.

"How long do I have?" I asked.

"Given what we know about your history and that you've probably had it for several years, maybe three or four years."

Three or four years, I thought.

"Shane, this is not an easy disease. You may start seeing some effects earlier."

I saw the anguish on his face.

A devout Christian and a faithful man, Dr. Kent quoted a few Scriptures to help ease the blow. But at the end of the conversation, the truth was still there: Unless something changed, I was not going to survive this, and it would not be an easy death either. The body basically turned on itself. It wasn't the HIV or AIDS that killed you; it was the myriad other diseases that infected your body that ultimately did you in — diseases with horrible names like Karposi's sarcoma and pneumocystis pneumonia. Of course, there were also dementia, blindness, loss of hearing, and finally, wasting. I was living with a monster of a disease inside me. I thought about Ryan White and the Ray family going through this ordeal. I had been thankful, even in prayer, that this disease had passed me by. But now here it was— inside me.

CONVERSATIONS

Dr. Kent had called my mom the day before, and they had decided it was time for me to know about my diagnosis. I was in a very serious dating relationship, and though Pokey and I had both been active in the "True Love Waits" program, Dr. Kent and my mom knew the power and uncertainty of teenage hormones. They also agreed that I had come a long way emotionally since the eye surgery, and it was time for me to take on this news for myself. I am not sure why Dr. Kent drew the duty of telling me, but while he was doing that, my mom was home keeping herself busy.

After I left the doctor's office, I went home and found my mom waiting. She had wondered how I would receive both the news of the disease and the idea that the information had been kept from me all of these months. This was in the days before cell phones, so there was no way to contact her or let her know. Thus she simply waited. When I walked in, she came over and gave me a huge hug and repeatedly said she was sorry for both the news and all of the months of not telling me. I assured her that I understood why they had remained silent, although part of me was shaken by the deception. I had trusted implicitly the adults in my life, and to take them at their word was just part of who I was. Although this trust changed forever that day, I also understood that we were in the big leagues in terms of important, explosive information, and no one had a rule book for how to handle the various issues that would arise around such a diagnosis.

We sat next to each other on the sofa, but neither of us said much. What was there to say? I could sense that we both wanted some time to let the information sink in. She could tell that I was processing what I had just been told, and I knew that she was trying to gauge how I had taken the news. She held my hand as we tried desperately not to let the other see the tears in our eyes. As usual, my mom was strong, but she seemed to be weary and confused as we sat together. She bore the weight of this news for months. And through holidays and other events during this time, she remained focused on what she thought was best for me. Of course, part of it was also shock. We had both wished for much more from life than this. I had been her pride and joy, and she had taken such good care of me. And for that, I had tried to be a good son, following the rules and making sure that I made her proud of me. But this moment on the sofa was difficult. We had weathered a lot together. I could tell she was crying, and that made me cry too. Finally, she reached her arms around me and drew me close. She kept whispering that things would be okay and that she would take care of me. I believed her. She had always taken care of me, from the scratches to the bruises to the major medical events. I knew she wouldn't fail me now.

Looking back on the scene now as a father and knowing how much my own children mean to me, I can only imagine how fearful my mother must have felt. Though neither of us dared say it, we felt as though the disease might be too big for even us to face. We just sat there and continued to hold each other. We were not prone to affection, and I don't remember many times since that we hugged like that. But I will always remember that moment.

I didn't know how to tell Pokey. Dr. Kent was especially concerned about Pokey, even as I assured him that we were not sexually active. The week I learned of my diagnosis, Pokey was visiting her father in Kentucky. How would she take the news? Most girls her age would have run at the first mention of the word. My last girlfriend before Pokey had once said that she would never want to be in the same room with a person who was HIV positive. Even though I knew that Pokey was different, I still feared that she would break up with me, and while I waited for her to come home, I prepared myself to lose her. Both Dr. Kent and Mom had said that it might be too much for Pokey to take and that I should, for her own good, let her out without much effort if I felt that it was what she needed. *What she needed*, I kept thinking. These felt like conversations for people so much older than us. But that was the world we were in now.

I remember thinking how unfair this all seemed. I was a good kid, or at least I tried to be, and this was not the way the plan was supposed to unfold. I didn't like the way it made my mother feel. I didn't like the fear, the prospect of what the disease would do to me. I didn't like the way it stole our present and our future from us. Every conversation and every relationship had to be thought out with great care. Now that I have told countless thousands of people about my condition, it is peculiar to think of the struggle of those initial conversations. But the 1980s were volatile, uncertain times for those diagnosed with HIV/AIDS.

Misinformation and fear made it more than simply difficult to speak with others; they made it dangerous.

CRADLED

When Pokey arrived home, we made plans to see each other the next day, which happened to be the Fourth of July. We attended a family picnic early in the day, but Pokey knew something was bothering me. I sensed the same thing from her. We were both on edge, and the day was tense.

Pokey and I sat down in her mom's sunlit living room, and after some hesitation, I told Pokey I had something important to say. She smiled nervously. Although Pokey liked to put on a tough demeanor, she could be very affectionate, and during hard conversations, she liked to draw physically close. As our discussion deepened, she could tell that I was struggling, and she had gotten so close to me that she was practically sitting in my lap. Having her in my life meant so much to me that the next words were the hardest I've ever spoken.

I told Pokey that I was HIV positive. It took several agonizing minutes for me to babble out my carefully prepared speech—I spoke about my transfusions, my eye surgery, the life expectancy for HIV/AIDS patients, the complications to our romantic future, the discrimination and stigma surrounding my disease, and my willingness to go along with whatever decision she made—but at last I finished. I needed to be strong and brave, I thought, but as my eyes filled with tears, I fell silent. Time crawled by as we sat together, and my grief ached like poison in my veins.

Then Pokey put her hand on my chin and turned my face

until I was looking at her. "I need to tell you a few things too," she said. "I'm not okay on the inside either, and there are some things you need to know before we go any further. I'm not who you think I am," she said softly. "But I'm not sure *I* know who I am anymore, either."

Pokey shared about her broken self-image, childhood sexual abuse, her battle with an eating disorder, an abusive former relationship, and her constant struggle to discover her identity.

I sat speechless, holding her hand, pulled out of myself by love.

"God put us together," she said. "I knew something was different when I met you."

I wrapped my arms around the person who had become my best friend and the love of my life. Neither of us had expected to find our "soul mates" at such an early age, no more than we had expected the bottom to fall out of our lives with all of this serious news. But as young as we were, our relationship felt deep and real — more mature by the second.

"Do you think you can love someone like me?" she asked.

"The real question is, do you think you can love someone like me?"

"I already do," she said.

We kissed, and it was gentle, sweet, and more intimate than anything I had ever known, our warm mouths confirming the truth of our words. I touched my forehead to hers, feeling her soft skin on mine. I could feel her heart beating as we remained for a long moment, touching. There was something powerful in touching and caressing someone you knew wanted to be that close to you. It was also at the heart of our fears that no one, because of the injuries and brokenness in each of us, would ever really want to touch us again. Not the way it mattered anyway. Who would want to be that close to an HIV positive kid? Who would want to be intimate and just hold and be close to a girl who had been touched by so many in inappropriate ways? The negative voices kept assaulting us, but the more they shouted, the more we held each other. I wiped the tears from Pokey's face, and she kissed me what seemed like a thousand times. Finally, we pulled back away from each other, realizing where this was heading and not wanting the confusion to get any more out of control.

"I'm not going anywhere," she said, tears tracing wet curves across her face.

I asked her to pray.

"Hey, God," she began softly.

"Hey, God," indeed. We were in God's hands. There was nothing we could do but trust in the One who had brought us together, two wounded teenagers sitting forehead to forehead on a sunlit couch, realizing that in the blink of an eye we had both grown up well beyond our years and that we were indeed in new waters. I would never touch her the same again, and she would never kiss me the same. We were in this for life, and no matter what, we understood each other and knew what God was doing.

As we stood up to leave, I put my hand on her cheek, allowing her face to rest in my hand for a moment. Her eyes closed again. I just stood there and looked at her. Even at sixteen, she was beautiful, with a grace and elegance that most women twice her age did not have. But I also knew the pain she held inside, and at that moment I so wanted to take it away from her — just as she wanted to take the pain from me. But we couldn't, and the best we had was to be with each other.

Chapter 3

THE SHALLOW WATER

*Today I became a Methodist, but I still don't think I will tell
my grandmother yet. My mother took it in stride. She knew
it was coming with me dating Pokey. But I didn't become a
Methodist because of Pokey. It is hard to convince everyone
of this, but I can see their point too. No, I like Wesley. Pretty
much everything about him—his theology, his tenacity, his
hope for the church. Listen to me ... I sound like a preacher.*

—Journal entry, July 16, 1989

assumed my health would decline rapidly. Others around me expected the same. Anticipating that each day might be the beginning of the end, my life took on a sense of urgency. My accelerated expectations and dreams caused restlessness. I faced life with a new determination and drive that would, in the future, be my greatest strength and weakness.

Pokey and I finished high school inseparable. The phrase "Pokey and Shane" became like one name, and people began to see us changing. Friends joked that I was dressing better and becoming interested in the culture and world around me, while Pokey began speaking up about important issues around school. She went, almost overnight, from being a hyper girl interested in homecoming festivities to a mature young woman working for community projects like Habitat for Humanity and the Humane Society. She also began asserting herself more in school activities and sharing her leadership abilities — by her senior year, she was elected president of her class, the student council, and the Beta Club, as well as editor of the annual.

I graduated from high school the year before Pokey. Unwilling to leave her side, I attended the Honors College of the University of Southern Mississippi in our hometown of Hattiesburg. Since no one knew about my health condition, everyone assumed I had a serious case of puppy love, which I did, but things were more complicated than that. Neither Pokey nor I wanted to waste any of our remaining time on a long-distance romance.

THE SHALLOW WATER

I grew up as a Southern Baptist, but my senior year of high school I started attending church with Pokey — a small United Methodist congregation in Hattiesburg. The pastor — a tall, thin man who reminded me of Ichabod Crane — tried to convert me from the beginning. "You would make a fine Methodist. You're short, smart, and a little boring. Perfect for the shallow water," he said. This was a reference to the way United Methodists baptize. Baptists believe that baptism is by immersion, while Methodists usually baptize by sprinkling water on the top of the head. In the old days, when most baptisms were done in rivers and creeks, the Baptists would gather in the deeper water, while the Methodists congregated in the shallow water near the shore.

Reverend Walley was a kind, soft-spoken man with tremendous people skills. We hit it off immediately, sharing a taste for dry humor and bad jokes. Reverend Walley saw something in me that I had never explored: the potential to become a preacher. After that first youth service, I had continued to preach, mostly in small churches or at youth events, but the idea of being a pastor had never crossed my mind. I had always planned on being a lawyer and was studying prelaw in college, but Reverend Walley saw differently. Through a series of very smooth arrangements, he offered me a part-time job as his assistant, and even as I continued to study law, I took on more and more pastoral duties.

KNOWING AND BEING KNOWN

I spent a year working for Reverend Walley, eventually joining the United Methodist Church as a member. I helped him develop a wonderful program of small groups long before small groups were the next big thing. I witnessed the importance of community dialogue in taking complete strangers and turning them into friends—and reducing potential conflict in the church along the way. It was hard to be mad at someone if you knew you had to pray for them at the same time, a point that would come in handy later.

Throughout the year, my health continued to be strong, though a series of blood work showed the first signs that my immune system was being affected by the disease. My T-cell count, the number used to indicate the body's immune system strength, was weakening. Dr. Kent, who had been following my condition in association with the hematology department at the University Medical Center in Jackson, suggested I see an Infectious Disease (ID) specialist. Since ID doctors weren't taking patients in Hattiesburg, my only option was to use a physician in Jackson.

I was ushered into a stark white room and told to strip, put on a gown, and wait. Pokey was made to wait outside. The doctor arrived with his nurse and began to poke and prod in very uncomfortable places.

After the exam, he prescribed AZT (azidothymidine, an antiviral drug that inhibits the replication of some retroviruses, such as HIV), reminded me to have safe sex, and told me to put my clothes on. He said there was little they could do except treat various symptoms. Given the length of time I'd already had the disease, I should expect a sharp decline in my health over the next months. He turned and left the room while the nurse handed me a slip of paper and told me to make my return appointment at the front desk. I never went back.

This was my first encounter with the difficulty of managing

the disease.* But most people with my condition encountered that type of story on a regular basis. For instance, the physical location of the clinic was located in the basement of the hospital. Officials said the location was due to a space issue only, but it required HIV/AIDS patients to go through a separate entrance, far away from the normal traffic flow. Even more isolating than the clinic location was the demeanor of the medical personnel who worked there. Many who worked in Infectious Disease were more interested in the science than in the people. More than anything, it was the emotional side of the disease that made care so complicated. We certainly needed scientists willing to gather data and work for new treatments, but people were dying in large numbers through extraordinarily difficult conditions, and they needed whole-patient care. My first visit was far from that, and I immediately felt the sting of what this disease meant for me and for so many to carry.

CLOUDY, SUNNY DAYS

Christmas is one of my favorite times of the year. Pokey and I always look forward to the festivities and to the sweet, gentle nature of the season. The distraction from our normal concerns is also nice. During Christmastime in 1989 I surprised Pokey by asking her to marry me and by giving her an engagement ring. We had talked about getting married from almost the day we started dating, and everyone assumed that eventually we would. But as we finished high school and entered college, we both became involved

---

*"Managing" may seem like an ordinary term, but that is exactly what you do when you discover you are HIV positive. You manage the physical effects, the medicines, and the emotional and relational impact. You "manage" it, or it will manage you.

in various activities, and I also started working for my father's printing business as a sales rep. It was a busy time. Thus, marriage had fallen off the radar for many people, including Pokey.

A week before Christmas, I made plans for us to go to dinner at one of the nicer restaurants in town. I had sold a large account the day before, and she assumed that the dinner was to celebrate the sale. After the meal was served, the waiter asked if he could get us dessert. I readily accepted (a rarity for me), and Pokey joined in. When the server arrived at the table with the Death by Chocolate dessert I had ordered along with a secret bottle of champagne, Pokey knew something was up — for a couple of reasons. One, champagne was very expensive, and we didn't have the money to spare. But we were also underage for drinking, and the server never asked for our ID.

The server poured two glasses of champagne. I took the ring out of my pocket, walked around the table, and knelt on one knee. "Pokey," I said, looking into her eyes, "we have been through a lot over these years, and you have been a beautiful, wonderful gift to my life." Pokey smiled, and tears began to form in her eyes. I stopped, handed her a tissue, and began again. "Would you do me the honor of making the rest of the journey with me as my wife?" I stopped and put the ring one-third of the way onto her finger, then asked, "Pokey, will you marry me?"

Pokey put her right hand over her mouth and then to her forehead as she began to cry. Finally, after what seemed like forever, she said, "Yes, I would love to be your wife." We had not realized that the rest of the diners had taken notice by this time and were watching. I reached up and kissed Pokey. Just then, the other patrons began to clap and cheer.

Everyone we knew was happy for us, including Pokey's

family. Over the years, her family had accepted me as one of their own. We had told Pokey's mother of my health not long after Pokey learned the news herself. And over the years, I would grow even more thankful for how Pokey's family faced my health concerns. Especially after having children myself, I realize the true blessing of her family being so willing to support us. Many families would not have been so willing. But Pokey's family could see, as young as we were, that we loved each other and that we certainly had not approached these issues blindly.

Most believed it would be a few years before we were married, or at least given any other circumstances for any other couple, it should have been. Those who knew us, however, realized the time constraints we faced. But we also had technical issues to deal with: I would lose my health insurance once I got married, so we both needed good jobs with benefits before we could be married. Therefore, we decided to be patient about setting a date. We believed that God would provide an opportunity for us to get good jobs, but we were both a couple of years away from graduating. The date, then, would be set after those issues were settled. But even though we knew our wedding might be long way off, we were elated about the engagement. Pokey was beautiful and giddy with everyone she told. I could tell she was happy. Goodness knows, I was.

New blood work showed that my immune system was weakening more quickly, raising a new level of urgency for us. This was the first time I truly felt the fear of what would happen to Pokey and me because of the disease. Since I was asymptomatic, we lived normally, but with my T-cell numbers dropping, the emotional effects were noticeable.

That spring I suffered my first and only bout with depression and physical anxiety. One evening at home in my apartment, I began to sweat and my heart raced. I didn't know it at the time, but I was having an anxiety attack. A few days earlier, I had bitten my tongue while chewing on a piece of candy. I didn't realize that I was continuing to bleed, and I had kissed Pokey several times throughout the evening. It was only when she tasted blood that I understood what had happened. Pokey had obviously ingested some of my blood. I knew that the odds were very low that Pokey was in danger, but something about that evening caught me off guard, and for the next several days, I began to worry about what Pokey and I were doing—how could I ask her to risk her life?

On the night of the anxiety attack, I sat in the corner most of the night crying and holding my Bible. I wasn't sure what was wrong with me. It was as if the walls were closing in, yet I couldn't even explain the real issue or what I was experiencing. All I knew was that the weight of our situation had hit me all at once. Several times the night before, I had awakened feeling tired and sad, as if someone had thrown a blanket on me and I couldn't find my way out. The feelings continued for the next few days. Trying to "snap out of it" didn't help either, as the circumstances seemed to compound the other emotions. I felt sad and angry and alone simultaneously. The thought of dying and leaving Pokey as a young widow or asking her to risk her own health by being intimate with me pushed in on me. We had dealt with all of these questions and details before. But this was heightened and very direct. I often felt like running out the door and not looking back. My depression became so serious that Pokey and I sought counseling. The issues crossed the spectrum from normal thoughts of grief to my future with Pokey and putting her health in jeopardy. My anxiety became so strong that I refused even to kiss Pokey, afraid that I might harm her. "No matter how sunny the day is," I told our therapist, "I always feel like it's about to storm."

The therapist helped us to frame for the first time what was real in this disease and what was not, and what we could control and what was beyond our powers. It was a very difficult time. Of course, no one knew what we were going through or the depth of my sadness as we confronted these issues. It was not the last time Pokey and I would face such problems while the rest of the world assumed everything was perfect. We were not asking for anything out of the ordinary, but we were also very hesitant to share our thoughts or feelings with anyone, even those in our Bible study groups. The ones who knew the immensity of our struggles, including our families, did their best to take care of us. But their care was limited, considering that even we didn't understand the full scope of what having this disease meant. And because others did not know about or understand the pressure we were under, we could not talk about it like others who might be going through difficult circumstances. Thus our relationships were often complicated and lacked real depth.

Furthermore, we had to deal with the constantly shifting sands of the disease with new meds on the horizon but still an increasing body count. And we shared in the pain as we heard more and more stories of discrimination and loss. This time in our lives was a complex emotional stew of normal angst for life-changing moments mixed with the details and complexities of, at the time, the world's newest form of leprosy. I lost my appetite and couldn't sleep. I struggled to talk with God. Life was not only emotionally painful, but physically too. I told people—the ones I talked to at all—that I felt as if I had the flu, but no medicine made me feel better. Each day was a battle.

I eventually came out of my depression, but not without a lot of help from our family therapist and the love and support of family and friends. It also took a lot of self-reflection, personal spiritual focus, and just plain, stubborn spiritual courage. One person in particular who prayed for me and Pokey would send daily reminders in the form of calls, notes, or cards about God's strength and presence. This friend believed, as I did, that this episode of my life was a direct spiritual attack. Of course, as depression does, it manifested itself in and through many different means in my life, including emotional, spiritual, relational, and physical symptoms. And though I have not experienced those intense feelings since, I certainly acknowledge their power to cause those who suffer from depression to feel their effects and, many times, consider themselves hopeless.

Feeling those feelings and thinking those thoughts taught me an invaluable lesson about the powerful impact and possibilities, both good and bad, of our emotions on the daily routine and success of our lives. I learned that we often surrender to the adversary much of our happiness and stability. Needless to say, this episode would dramatically impact my ministry and my sensitivities for others who deal with similar issues.

LITTLE PREACHER BOY

The local district superintendent of the United Methodist Church in our area asked if I would be interested in serving as the pastor of a small church in a neighboring community. The congregation averaged fewer than fifty worshipers on Sundays and was mainly older individuals. The congregation seemed to be in its final days, having failed to welcome new and more diverse people into its fellowship. It had begrudgingly watched the surrounding community change demographically. The district superintendent made no bones about the fact that my job was to help this older congregation die with dignity, so that a newer congregation could emerge with a more open approach to ministry. The UMC leadership had given up on change; they decided, instead, to wait for this congregation to die or move away. Not exactly a church growth strategy.

The district superintendent appointed me as pastor at Justice Heights in June. The position provided a small salary, housing, and, most important, health benefits for both of us. Pokey and I were ready to set a date for a wedding. Between our emotional struggles in the spring and my dropping T-cell count, our families understood the rush. We set the date for August 18, 1990.

In June I moved into the large parsonage at Justice Heights. During my first week, my bicycle was stolen and one of the neighborhood children threw a rock through my window. Not only did the front door have a dead bolt, but so did the bedroom door — the result of a break-in that had taken place during the tenure of a previous pastor. It was a shock from the quiet apartment where I had been living.

However, the people in the congregation and my neighbors were very kind and excited about this young pastor and his soon-to-be wife. They took us in and treated us as their own. They even gave me the nickname "Little Preacher Boy."

This was the first time in my life I realized the importance of "place." One of the most destabilizing effects of chronic or serious illness is the sense of being "lost" around people you know. When we are sick, grieving, or lost, our "placed-ness" can shatter, sending sharp fragments flying into every aspect of our lives. Justice Heights restored my sense of place. It anchored me for a time. God has created us to root ourselves in places, because in places we find relationships with the people who live there. When we live faithfully in a place, at the service of our neighbors, the fullness of God's love can shine through. Justice Heights was the first place we experienced this, but it wouldn't be the last.

LESSONS AND LIFE AS PRETTY AS A PICTURE

As our wedding day drew near, Pokey and I attended the normal premarital classes, but unbeknownst to everyone else, we were also enrolled in another set of classes, talking with Dr. Kent about deeper emotional and physical issues of intimacy. We wouldn't have the luxury of making any mistakes.

We understood that the only entirely safe way of living was abstinence, but neither of us wanted that. However, we wanted to be as safe as reasonably possible. This included knowing not only the best practices for safe sex, but also understanding that consistency in our methods was important. Of course, this required planning and took some of the spontaneity out of intimacy, which led to the feeling in our conversations that intimacy lacked a certain emotional quality. Getting around this was a concern.

I was particularly concerned about the emotional context of our intimacy. I found it difficult to accept that making love to my wife — no matter how safe we were — would put at risk the person I loved most. I faced issues of pride as well: Could I "be the man" my wife deserved, even with all our precautions and planning? Pokey never even hinted that she was concerned about this, but it remained on my mind. If Pokey wasn't "in the mood" — a normal enough occurrence in any relationship — would I interpret that in light of my disease?

Dr. Kent helped us see that everything in our relationship needed to be framed in a new context because of my disease. Although much of our life together would be as normal as any couple's, we would always need to be aware of the crucial differences.

Pokey and I were married in a beautiful ceremony at an outdoor worship center near our home. Since the small worship area was built in the middle of the woods, only fifty people could attend.

Jason, my best friend since third grade, served as my best man. I told Jason my HIV status at the rehearsal dinner, years after he broached the subject of the disease while we played water volleyball as sixth graders. At first, he simply looked at the ground; I couldn't tell what he was feeling. Finally, Jason looked up with tears in his eyes. He said he had thought about the issue several times over the years but had never asked.

"Are you okay?" I asked.

"Yes," he said, looking down. Jason is brilliant and never at a loss for words. We had spent a great deal of time together as kids and throughout our teenage years. I knew this news was not a complete shock to him, but I could also imagine what it meant for him to hear it now. Was he scared? Was he angry that I had not told him sooner? Was he upset and grieved for me? Was it all of the above?

He had said yes, but I wasn't sure if he meant it.

"Just give me a few seconds," he said. We were standing in the breezeway outside of the fellowship center where we had dinner. I patted him on the shoulder and walked past him to give him his space.

Several minutes later, he reappeared at the festivities with his customary smile. He walked over and told one of his notoriously bad jokes. As everyone scattered back into their other groups, I made eye contact with him. He smiled and gave me a wink. I knew we would be okay.

The next day at 6:00 p.m. I stood at the front of the outdoor chapel, my hands dripping sweat like a faucet. As nervous as I've ever been, I kept reminding myself not to lock my knees — though I was so nervous I didn't even remember *why* I was telling myself that!

The setting was beautiful — a brick, open-air chapel with wood beams and pews that gave it both a natural but also reverent feel. The tall pines that surrounded the worship area and the creek that ran just behind the chancel area made for as beautiful a setting as one could imagine. But all that paled when Pokey made her way down the aisle, her grandfather on one arm and her great-grandfather on the other. When I saw her, I was literally unable to breathe. Her elegant, cream-colored dress seemed to sway in time with the beat of my heart; the flowers she had scattered provided a makeshift rug; and the rays of light coming through the trees shone on her radiant face.

By the time Pokey reached the altar, she was crying. Her back to our gathered friends and family, she whispered to me out of the side of her mouth. "Is my makeup running?"

I laughed and then put my hand on her cheek to wipe away her tears, all the while thinking about what it had cost us just to get to this day. Who would have imagined that the couple sharing a seat on the school van all those years ago would have ended up here?

I felt blessed and awed. The minister started the ceremony, but it wasn't until it was time for me to answer the vows—helped by an elbow from Pokey—that I paid attention to anything but her. I blurted out, "Yes ... I do!" and we moved on from there. The rest of the ceremony is a blur. This was our moment, and for once we didn't feel the need to explain anything or put anything "into perspective." We had worried, wondered, and prayed, but this was our time to celebrate, no matter what we faced.

The only downside to the day was the outfit that Pokey picked out for me. She wanted us to match—it's a Southern thing—and my outfit included a hideous pair of purple shorts, a purple and white shirt, and purple socks. I looked, frankly, unbelievably ugly, and I've since hidden all of the pictures. My aunt declared the whole day to be as "pretty as a picture," and I agree.

Except for that outfit.

HONEYMOON HITCHES

When Pokey first read what I'm about to share with you, she said, "Shane, no one wants to know about our honeymoon." I replied, "Yes, but I want to talk about it." To that she responded, "Men!"

And thus, by the time you read this, I'll be sleeping on the sofa and wondering why there is one less place setting at the table. I hope it's worth it.

We spent our first night as husband and wife in a beautiful bed and breakfast a couple of hours from our home. We rushed into our room together—I was anxious to proceed with what I called the "normal honeymoon activities," while Pokey later admitted that she was more interested in the snacks her brides- maids had cached for us. And now I can admit: the food was great too.

After all of our conversations, counseling, and concerns, the moment turned out more real and genuine than either of us could have dreamed. We did everything we were supposed to do from a medical standpoint, but the look in Pokey's eyes and the touch of her skin made the moment transcendent. We lay in each other's arms and knew that we had committed every part of ourselves to one another. Our long journey had been well worth it. After we made love, though, Pokey started crying. Honestly, I thought I had done something wrong and asked if everything was okay.

"It was perfect," she said, tears still rolling down her cheeks. "I have just never felt so beautiful and special before." Physi- cal intimacy, for an abuse survivor, is an assault on self-esteem and self-image. I wasn't the only broken person being healed as grace transformed our present and gave us a glimpse of our bright future. To this day, about twenty years later, I still love to be close to Pokey, the touch of her skin and the sweet sound of her voice close to me. No matter what has happened in our marriage, that kind of intimacy has never lost importance for us. The experience goes much deeper than just sex or the physical response, because to each of us, being close in that way symbol- izes so much more—namely, acceptance and affirmation.

The rest of the honeymoon was equally wonderful, but if I stop now, I may just be allowed off the couch and back into bed with Pokey!

The next two years were some of the best of our lives. We settled into a routine, attending school and working at Justice Heights. Pokey served as children's director, counselor, hostess, and a hundred other things, and I continued to work part-time for my father's printing business. Pokey also opened a dance studio in our poor neighborhood. The job cost us more money than we made — our extra funds went to buy clothes, dance costumes, and basic supplies for the kids — but the smiles on the kids' faces as they discovered the art in their bodies was priceless.

Our church was small but was filled with great joy and fellowship. The church began reaching beyond the block into the housing projects next door. We donated old Bibles to the local Boys & Girls Club that had set up shop in the project's community center. Members of one of the women's Sunday school classes provided refreshments for the after-school program and supplies for the arts and crafts classes. Our neighbors were no longer "those people" but became acquaintances and then friends. The shift didn't happen overnight, but member after member became connected to the place and people we all called home.

By the second year of our tenure, more than half of us were involved in responding to the needs of the surrounding community and housing project. For our efforts, the members of Justice Heights were named Small Membership Church of the Year by the local Methodist conference. The members, like Pokey and me, had discovered the joy of place, forging relationships that continued even after the church closed several years later.

Chapter 4

T CELLS AND THRESHOLDS

I just stood in front of the chapel [at Duke University] and felt like I belonged there. I am still worried about moving so far away, though. My T-cell count is below 50, and sometimes I think moving so far away from home is crazy. What happens if I get sick?... Oh, if people knew what we were dealing with! But they don't, so I will be quiet and stop whining now.

—Journal entry, March 28, 1992

Reaching past the pines and rich hardwoods of Durham, North Carolina, are the spires of Duke Chapel. From the first moment I saw the Gothic architecture of Duke University's West Campus chapel, I felt like I was home.

Standing nearly 210 feet tall and seating well over eighteen hundred people, it is a most impressive structure. It is also a moral voice and constant reminder that the university, no matter how secular its reputation, has distinct ties to the United Methodist Church.

Reverend Walley convinced me to look into Duke Divinity School when I began to think about theology instead of law as a career. The previous year I had pastored Justice Heights, attended a few classes at a local nondenominational seminary, and waited for Pokey to graduate from college. I felt called to professional ministry, though I wasn't always happy about that call!

I enjoyed being involved in solutions for people and communities, and I cherished those moments people reserve only for their pastor, or someone similar, when they lower their guard and share from the core of their hearts. Of course, there is much about the job that I didn't (and still don't) like. Yet I saw the potential for the true transformation that can happen through the body of Christ.

Over the course of that year, I completed the candidacy program for ministry in the United Methodist Church and informed the local officials of my desire to enter into full-time ministry. The process was simple and without much fanfare. I filled out a few forms, completed a short guidebook about ministry and the life of a minister, and then appeared before the district Board of Ordained Ministry. The board asked a series of questions about my background, my ministry at Justice Heights, and my future plans. They seemed pleased with my intentions. No one asked about my health—in hindsight I wonder what would have happened differently if I had mentioned that I was HIV positive—and I was under no obligation to disclose my whole health background. The United Methodist Church was in need of committed young pastors, especially those who were not afraid of public speaking, so it seemed as though we were a fitting match. My time at Justice Heights had gone very well, so everyone seemed excited about my future in the church.

Pokey and I were concerned about the huge changes in our lives that moving to Duke would require. My T-cell count had continued to decline over the previous months, and I had still not found a doctor to follow my HIV. I also needed a job, and I sorted fruitlessly through staff listings at larger churches or in "field placements"—missional opportunities at various parachurch agencies. As the date for committing to the next semester at Duke drew closer, we questioned God's plan for our move. Naturally our anxiety rose. We certainly believed that I was called to ministry and Duke was the place, but was this the right time for moving?

Finally, an older gentleman at Justice Heights, who could tell that we were worried about next steps, sat us down one Sunday evening and asked if we were okay. We were not. At all.

"Do you believe God wants what is best for you?" he asked.

"Yes."

"Do you believe you can trust his leading?" he asked.

"Yes," we affirmed.

"What do you believe God is calling you to do in the next stages of your journey?" he asked.

"We believe he is leading us to attend graduate school," Pokey said.

"Then what's the holdup?" he asked. "It doesn't appear to be God."

He was right. The holdup was most certainly us. But we needed confirmation, so our friend challenged us to try something.

"Have you ever thrown out a fleece and watched for God to work?" he asked.

Fleece? Where had I heard that before? I was vaguely familiar with the story of Gideon. He had tested God, and because of Gideon's heart, God had answered him not once but two times.

I struggled with the theology of it. *Didn't Jesus say not to tempt the Lord your God? But wait, this isn't temptation or testing; this is about clarity. But isn't it like a test? This is too confusing.* We debated for several days about the appropriateness and the process of how to "throw out a fleece." Finally, after running out of other options, we decided our fleece would bring together two of the most sacred institutions on the planet — the church and the U.S. Postal Service.

One of our friends had grown tired of our hemming and hawing, so she suggested the following plan: On Monday, if we received something in the mail from Duke, the deal was sealed. We had been receiving a lot of info lately, so this didn't seem like a major test, but it was worth a try.

Sure enough, on Monday I walked to the mailbox and found a housing brochure sent from the admissions office of Duke about possible accommodations. We had received mail out of the blue before from Duke, but this was certainly a good start. Like good, faithful Gideons, we threw a second fleece. On Tuesday, if we received information about financial aid from the school, we would consider this God's leading. In the mail Tuesday was a pamphlet, hand-signed by the director of admissions, about ministerial education funds available to entering students from Mississippi.

Now we were paying attention. Two fleeces, two answers. But we decided that twice was not enough. We threw a third fleece, one with a little muscle behind it. We needed a job. So on Wednesday we would need information from the director of admissions about possible job openings or pastoral appointments. We were afraid to mention the whole scenario out loud; after all, we were playing games with the God of the universe, and he was winning.

On Wednesday we did not run to the mailbox. Instead, we both piddled around the house, neither wanting to be the first to look, although deep down we both wanted to make a mad dash for it. Finally, we caught each other's eyes and began to laugh. We opened the mailbox together: there was a letter from the admissions office about field placement opportunities, and in a handwritten note, the secretary had put on a separate piece of paper the numbers of the district superintendent of the Raleigh district as well as several other numbers of local churches. Most beautiful of all, in the bottom righthand corner, circled in red ink, was the name of one church, Benson Memorial UMC in Raleigh, which was looking for an assistant pastor and program director. Beside the position description was a handwritten note: "Thought this one might interest you."

As we read the note, our eyes filled with tears. God had answered our questions with patience and joy, reminding us that God's intentions for us are always in our best interest and for our own good—though clearly that may look different than we imagine. Pokey and I both felt silly about testing God with the U.S. Postal Service, but we certainly found peace in the answer. Sometimes our fragile spirits need a little help and a reminder to trust even what we cannot see.

The next day, I called the Divinity School of Duke University and accepted their invitation to attend classes.

NANCY

The other issue with which we struggled was our continued search for a physician to follow my HIV. Although more and more physicians were seeing patients living with HIV, the level of professional knowledge remained dishearteningly low. For many, seeing HIV/AIDS patients remained a difficult choice, especially in smaller communities. Adding to this dilemma was the fact that HIV was a medical nightmare when it came to the level, scope, and time of care involved. It was a difficult disease to manage that required a significant investment by the physician, and it also required a tremendous amount of specialized knowledge. Many people living with HIV found few doctors both willing and able to care for them.

Thankfully, though, the issue of HIV was moving out of the shadows from sermons about "lifestyle" and "morality" and into discussions about care and compassion. Ryan White helped provide a new face for the disease, as did Elizabeth Glaser, wife of actor Brian Glaser. Elizabeth contracted the disease through a blood transfusion and, tragically, passed the disease to her children. Elizabeth, Ryan, and countless other people living with HIV/AIDS fought to broaden the country's understanding of the disease. Without their efforts and the unwavering commitment of the gay and lesbian communities, many advancements related to treating the disease would not have taken place.

On November 8, 1991, a giant stride was taken toward public understanding of HIV/AIDS when basketball great Ervin "Magic" Johnson disclosed that he had tested positive for HIV. I was shocked and relieved. Magic Johnson was the first heterosexual sports figure to disclose his HIV status at the height of his career. Although tragic, his announcement was critical for the HIV community. Overnight Magic Johnson brought the discussion of HIV/AIDS into living rooms across the country.

Magic Johnson's infection galvanized the mainstream public to respond to the growing risk of HIV/AIDS. In turn, it also spurred increased research and development opportunities that resulted in a stream of new medicines and treatments. Prior to 1991, few treatments existed for fighting the disease. The first was AZT.*

Overnight, the conversation about HIV/AIDS changed

---

*Approved in 1987, AZT (azidothymidine or zidovudine) helped fight, albeit briefly, falling T-cell (CD4) counts. A T-cell is a type of white blood cell that matures in the thymus and carries out the cell-mediated immune response. There are three major types of T-cells: helper (CD4) T-cells, suppressor (CD8) T-cells, and killer (CD8) T-cells (cytotoxic T-lymphocytes, or CTLs). A dropping CD4 count indicates increased damage to the body's ability to respond to disease. This was and is the modus operandi of HIV. Normal CD4 counts run close to 1,000. Any number below 200 is considered, as defined by the Centers for Disease Control, as full-blown AIDS.

because of Magic Johnson. People began to talk more about individuals with HIV/AIDS with whom they had contact or about families who had been impacted by it. Prior to Magic Johnson's disclosure, I never had a single conversation about the disease, even with those who knew of my health condition. That is one of the reasons why locating a physician was so difficult.

Part of the reason no one talked about HIV/AIDS was because it was so highly stigmatized as a condition of those who had done something inappropriate or immoral. It was seen by so many as a gay man's disease or as the disease of malcontents. So even with the "innocent" victims (and I hate that phrase), people did not know how to have the conversations.

Second, there was little hope in those days for people who contracted the disease. People were dying, not living with HIV/AIDS, and even the ones who contracted the disease in more "acceptable" ways, did not have a particularly good prognosis.

Therefore, HIV/AIDS communities either existed as militant or underground. In mainstream midsized communities, it was difficult to find the local support groups (if there was one) or anyone who could tell of other available resources, except for a few social workers at the health department.

Given all of this, one could understand why a family doctor in a smaller community might not advertise that he or she was seeing HIV/AIDS patients. As a person once told me while standing in line, just seeing "those folks" in the waiting room made people feel uncomfortable.

In the early winter of 1992, my dentist told me of a doctor in an adjacent town who had been seeing HIV patients for several years. Dr. Nancy Tatum, a former high school music teacher, worked with her father in a small family practice clinic. Dr.

Tatum started seeing HIV patients by accident. She was called into the emergency room at the local hospital several years earlier to treat a former high school student who was showing signs of an unusual type of pneumonia. The young man had recently moved home from another state after several months of a prolonged illness. Nancy quickly realized that the illness was AIDS and that his pneumonia was one of the opportunistic infections. She remembers how, after seeing her former student, she went immediately to the restroom and scrubbed herself from head to toe. Even for medical professionals, the early days of HIV/AIDS were uncertain.

Word spread, usually through clandestine channels, that Nancy was seeing those infected with HIV/AIDS. By the time we met, nearly 150 HIV positive patients were being treated at Nancy's clinic.

Nancy was something of a kickback to the small town doctors of the 1940s and '50s. Her clinic, off of Main Street in the little town of Petal, Mississippi, was an older, ranch-style house that smelled of cleaning supplies and rubbing alcohol. Visiting the clinic reminded me of an episode straight out of the 1970s classic TV show, *Marcus Welby, M.D.*, where the cases were simple, though oftentimes emotional, and there was always a happy ending. Of course, that was not the case for many of Nancy's patients, but her loving demeanor made it seem possible.

Nancy's optimistic smile and relaxed attitude promoted a calm atmosphere in her office. I realized immediately that Nancy was more than just a doctor for her patients; she was also a friend and an advocate. I made my first appointment with her in March 1992. I remember going through my explanation of why I needed to make an appointment, using all of the old verbiage of half explanation and half secrecy to try to paint a clear enough picture for the receptionist. I had been seeing other family physicians to cover my basic medical needs, and it was always daunting to walk in and announce that I was HIV positive. Most front desk personnel would ask why I needed to see the doctor. "I'm sick" never seemed to cover it, and as soon as the letters HIV came out of my mouth, strange looks crossed their faces. I had created lots of ways to say HIV without actually mouthing the words and to describe HIV as an add-on concern when presenting another problem or issue. And don't get me started about the new patient form on which I had to give my medical history. I actually heard one receptionist burst out with "Oh my God!" when she, obviously, read the diagnosis on the form. Needless to say, we did not go back to that clinic.

Nancy's clinic was very different. Finally, the receptionist, who was more than aware of what I was trying to say and what I needed, finally said, "Honey, you don't need to explain anything else. Dr. Tatum will be happy to see you." I can't explain what a relief this simple process was for someone in my condition.

My first visit was like a long sigh that relieved the pressure of months of anxiety and uncertainty. Although an excellent physician, Nancy's greatest gifts were her presence and the affirmation of her willingness to support her patients in the often painful, debilitating journey that AIDS exacted. A lifelong Methodist and committed Christian, she was nothing short of a miracle to me after my months of wondering what direction to go medically and constantly worrying about the turns and twists the next blood count would bring.

Those first months of our doctor-patient relationship, Nancy stabilized both my medical and emotional approach to the disease. She helped me mature as a person living with HIV and showed me how I could help others by sharing my story, albeit privately in those days. The fear of facing the disease head-on was replaced with a quiet determination to fight and with a hope for what tomorrow could bring. One of Nancy's valued services to her many patients was to continuously update us on the newest medical breakthroughs. She could turn the news of new medicines into a reason for celebration, even though for many it would be too late or the side effects would prevent any real benefit. "You are all going to outlive me" was her constant encouragement.

As I prepared to move to North Carolina, Nancy helped me locate physicians to care not only for my HIV but also for my hemophilia and eye problems. Her care as a physician and as a friend changed my life. She taught me about life and about faith from a perspective that no church or theologian could. Nancy reminded me of how powerfully the body of Christ can bring healing and testify to God's goodness. Nancy was, to so many, Christ. She touched the untouchable and loved the unloved. She was and remains the best example of Jesus that I have ever known.

That summer Pokey and I said good-bye to Mississippi, our families, and Justice Heights. We moved to North Carolina where Pokey found a job teaching in a school district an hour north of our new home. I worked at Benson Memorial UMC, a church that sat at the geographic center of the Raleigh community, as director of programs. Both of us worked on our graduate degrees. Pokey, who had finished her bachelor's degree in education, was pursuing a master's degree in education at a small liberal arts college.

As we drove into the Triangle area—the name the locals have for the cities of Raleigh, Durham, and Chapel Hill—we saw the spires of Duke Chapel. I thought about the way that its height reminded everyone of its constant presence. We felt the same way about God in our lives. We had moved far from home and the odds were stacked against us, but we knew where our strength came from, and we knew where to look. In the years to come, there would be times when we would lose ourselves, but like looking up and seeing the spires of Duke Chapel, we would never lose sight of God.

We arrived late that first day in Raleigh and drove to our new apartment. We had rented in the center of the vibrant, cultured town. As we approached the door, I unlocked it but told Pokey to stop.

"There's something I need to do," I said. I put my arms down around her to pick her up.

"What are you doing?"

"I am carrying you across the threshold! I may have missed it the first time, but never again." I grinned. "Every new adventure will begin like this."

"You mean with a pulled muscle in your back," she shot back, smiling.

"You don't think I can do it, do you?"

"I love you for trying! How's that?" she replied.

Without another word, I picked her up and moved across the threshold and into our new life. Our years in North Carolina would be some of the best of our marriage. The friendships and experiences remain with us to this day. But they would also be the years when my health would become about more than simply my physical condition. God had plans to carry us across life-changing thresholds that would make us laugh and cry and wonder beyond anything we could have imagined.

Chapter 5

PUTTING OUR FUTURE WHERE OUR FAITH IS

It feels like a new beginning. I keep praying we have made the right decision. I guess we are putting our lives where our faith is—just made that up. Okay, so I will never be a writer.

—Journal entry, June 1992

Within the first few months, despite homesickness, we settled into life with new friends, jobs, church, and schools. The church where I served embraced us immediately, and many people became lifelong friends. My job as assistant minister included ministry to young couples. Pokey and I, ages twenty-two and twenty-three respectively, were the youngest of the young couples. We named our new Sunday school class "The Thrillseekers" because we were thrilled to seek the will of God. We didn't mind that the rest of the congregation looked at us with mild suspicion. Most of the two dozen couples were transplants to the area, and the class became our family away from home.

I loved this group, and they were the first significant group of people who had no prior connection to me to whom I told of my condition. They were the first people to whom I laid open my life and simply trusted. My relationships with these friends showed me that no matter our circumstances, the power of community to build us from deep within and enable us to surpass what normally would define us is profound. If it had not been for these relationships, I am afraid that the circumstances surrounding my upcoming ordination might have overwhelmed us. But this group became our family away from family, our home away from home, and showed once and for all what the church could be when we simply acted like it.

The pastor and the church went out of their way to make us

comfortable. I assisted in worship every Sunday and preached on a regular basis. I told Hugh, the pastor, about my health soon after I arrived; he was one of the few people outside my family who knew I was HIV positive. His response was encouraging, and he committed to support us in any way he could. Others on staff and in the church also took us under their wings, and there were few weeks that we were not sharing a meal at someone's home. Though I had already pastored for several years, I was still only twenty-three, and many within the church felt the need to provide surrogate parenting for us. As homesick as we were, we didn't mind at all.

My health remained fairly strong, even though according to the standards of the Centers for Disease Control my T-cell count — below 200 — meant I had full-blown AIDS. I had found a wonderful doctor who watched after my HIV and daily routine of medical concerns. A variety of new medicines were released during this time, and I tried each of them. I discovered allergies to sulfa and other drugs that significantly reduced my choices for drug cocktail regimens. Medicines and their side effects have impacted me more than the effects of HIV/AIDS itself. The drugs were wonderful, but they came at a price, and we learned that each new discovery did not necessarily mean that I would be able to take them or that they would affect my course of the disease. Some of the drugs cause side effects similar to having the flu, every day, seven days a week. Others cause drowsiness; some cause anxiety. Most, if not all, cause diarrhea and upset stomach. HIV was a powerful, cunning disease that required a variety of tactics to fight. For the most part, each new drug impacted the course of the disease, especially the class called protease inhibitors discovered around the mid-1990s. But the side effects could be as deadly and as difficult as the disease itself. Thus, locating a cocktail that brought down the viral load, raised the T-cell count, and kept at bay certain symptoms of opportunistic infections was one thing. Finding a regimen that I could actually take on a daily basis was quite another. I learned then that it was not necessarily the drugs I had available, but the drugs I could take that determined my chance for success.

During my second year of seminary, I began the first phases of ordination as an elder in the United Methodist Church. The process for ordination as a United Methodist is complicated. Between candidacy, theology school, and probationary periods, it can take nearly seven years to complete. The first step is candidacy, which I finished prior to attending Duke. As my theological training continued, I would have a series of interviews to complete and papers to write. Every potential ordinand is assigned an interview team from the local conference's Board of Ministry—people charged with the process for ordaining a person into ministry. This team, clergy and lay alike, are assigned to interview the candidate, review the candidate's materials portfolio, and approve his or her "ordination papers" (a written document of several theological and ministry-related questions). These men and women face a difficult task, balancing the need to make a good decision for the church with providing encouragement and support for the ordinands.

I completed my preordination requirements and was scheduled to meet with the interview team on a trip home to Mississippi during the Christmas holidays. At that time in the United Methodist Church, clergy experienced two ordinations, the first as a deacon (as a means of preparing for ministry), and then, after a two-year probationary period, as an elder. Each of these ordinations was critical, not just because of its theological importance, but because it meant several things for the relationship of a person with his or her annual conference and the United Methodist Church. Persons who were ordained and in good standing were appointed to a local congregation or ministry and were eligible for the full benefits of the church—including health insurance, a pension plan, and death benefits for all surviving immediate family members.

Health and psychological reviews are a standard part of the ordination process, and I received a health form from the Board of Ministry asking my doctor to verify that I was in good health and available for appointment—and, by extension, for ordination. To our knowledge, up to that time, no board had ever dealt with an HIV positive person's appointment in a local church. The health form caught me off guard. I was not prepared for the process, not because I was trying to conceal my health status, but because the issue had always been private and I had always chosen when and where to reveal my status.

Mike Hicks is a tall, affable fellow with a calm demeanor who served as registrar of the Board of Ministry. There is probably no more thankless job in the church hierarchy than this position, which usually becomes a "problem catcher" for bad attitudes, lost papers, and myriad excuses about why documents are not turned in on time. Mike was the first to hear about my health condition, and he was clearly shaken by the news. His silence shook me too. Within a few minutes, Mike regained composure and advised me to complete the form and send it to him as soon as possible. He finished our conversation by saying he believed everything would turn out okay. I am not sure if he actually believed that, but I appreciated his optimism.

My doctor completed the form, and we mailed it to the registrar's office in Mississippi. I had finished my ordination papers a few weeks earlier. As I put the packet together in the large manila envelope to mail, I felt confident about every aspect of my theological work for ordination. Now the entire process hung on the response to my health issues.

Word spread fast through the Board of Ministry about my condition. The bishop of the Mississippi annual conference, Marshall L. Meadors, enlisted the help of his own physician, our own Nancy Tatum, who had moved to Jackson following her internship at Vanderbilt. Other strangers on the committee took a special interest in my situation, including a pastor named Rocky Miskelly. Rocky, who would later become a dear friend in ministry, was energetic and brilliant and advocated for me.

Unknown to me, I became the subject of phone conversations and special meetings. The issues at hand included not only my health, but also the question of appointability and health insurance cost, including, especially, the death benefit Pokey would receive if I were to die. The death benefits are one of the most important "perks" of ministry in the United Methodist Church. They provide generous assistance to the spouses and dependents of ordained ministers in the case of death or disability. This can be expensive, and members of the Board of Ministry knew very well what the numbers might be in my case, given my illness and Pokey's young age. One member of the board had done the math, and he had calculated that Pokey could potentially receive death benefits for nearly seventy years. This same member would famously say about me in a meeting, "He may be the only person who will be more expensive dead than alive."

My ordination soon became part of a wider debate among

liberal and conservative forces within the annual conference. I was the focal point and the first real opportunity that many of these people had to discuss larger issues about clergy compensation, benefits, and even the nature of calling and accountability. Thus, the process, almost overnight, became complex and layered with many issues — some about me, others not.

Finally, the chair of the Board of Ministry at the time, Larry Goodpaster (yes, that's his real name), realized the potential for my issue to spin out of control and become unmanageable. He charged the interview team assigned to me with the task of first answering the questions of "theological preparedness and call." If I wasn't called or ready for ministry, then the other issues wouldn't matter. With this decision, Reverend Goodpaster changed the dynamic of my ordination process and probably saved my ministry by redirecting the conversation.

Following the Christmas holidays, Pokey returned home to North Carolina while I stayed with my parents and prepared for the meeting with the ordination interview team. I arrived at the interview meeting with more than the normal angst of most ordinands. The process was stressful for anyone, but especially for me, given the complexity of my health issues. I did not know what I was walking into or who would be involved — that information was secret. What I did know was that a group of seven or eight men and women had spent the better part of the previous weeks looking over my deepest thoughts, deciding my theological health and predisposition for ministry, and then also developing questions about my physical health and how it would affect my ministry.

Driving up to the building, which was located at a Christian retreat center in a very rural area, I remember the first feelings of anxiety, of wanting to say the right things. I registered at the front desk, and the receptionist told me to wait in the lobby area. The chair of my interview team would come get me when they were ready.

Moments later the door opened and out stepped a tall, very attractive woman with long red hair and an infectious smile.

"My name is Vicki Loflin Gary," the woman said.

Vicki Gary had a reputation as a promising pastor in our annual conference. She could preach and was incredibly bright and articulate. I also learned from friends that she had the reputation of being sympathetic to causes of social justice. It never hurt, I thought, to do my homework. Vicki was also the daughter of a notable older pastor and thus knew the way the ordination game was played in church politics. Her father had championed many of the social justice causes and efforts of the past couple of decades, and so I was relieved to know that my interview chair would have grown up hearing about fairness and process.

"We've been looking forward to meeting you," she said. She had a playful smile on her face, and I could tell that she wanted to make me feel as much at ease as possible. But she also didn't want to pretend that we didn't have significant issues before us. I immediately felt better and followed her down a long hall to the interview room.

"I read your ordination papers," she said, making conversation. "Some members of our committee think they are the best since Lovett Weems." Weems was a Mississippi native who had become president of St. Paul's School of Theology, one of our official United Methodist seminaries, and was well respected in Methodist circles.

"I don't know what to say," I replied.

"I am not sure I agree with them," she said, looking over at me with another smile. I smiled back.

We walked into the interview room. Others on the interview team rose from around the U-shaped table, and I introduced myself to each one, shaking hands. Everyone was very polite, but there was an air of caution in the room. I could tell that this group had spent a great deal of time talking about my issues.

The first questions were about my theology and call to ministry. The committee seemed more than pleased with my answers, and we had a great discussion about how I viewed ministry and the life of the church. We also spoke about the theological differences between Methodists and Baptists, and our conversation went into such depth that many of us almost forgot that other issue before us.

Finally, someone asked the question. "Shane, tell us about your health and how you see this issue affecting your ministry and ability to pastor a church." I was glad it was out in the open, and I liked the way the question was phrased. It was not accusatorial or antagonistic, but a genuine question about ministry effectiveness.

"Well, to think that my health will not be an issue is naive," I said. Several around the table chuckled. I smiled. "But it is no different than anyone who has a health problem or physical disability. There will be precautions and considerations, but I plan to do everything in my power to take care of myself and to work hard wherever I am appointed."

The words felt good to say. For the first time, I was talking openly about my health. Several members asked follow-up questions, but they were mostly about their concern for me and the demands and strains ministry often places on a person. "Like anyone," I responded, "I will need to take care of myself and be realistic as to what I can accomplish. If you let it, ministry can kill you, no matter what diseases you have." Everyone around the table agreed.

"You might be the first person in the United Methodist Church to have dealt with this situation, but you most certainly will not be the last," one member of the interview team said. "You are setting an important precedent not only for HIV positive people but for anyone who struggles with a health issue." Over the past days, I had come to know the importance of the conversation for me and for the entire United Methodist Church. "But," the team member continued, "it is a conversation that is well overdue."

"Besides," one member continued, "the church grows best from good challenges."

We all laughed nervously.

I left the interview believing that I had just cleared the last hurdle before being ordained, but I soon discovered that a difficult course still stretched out in front of me.

SECRET MEETINGS

The interview team said that I should hear something in the next few weeks. So when I arrived home from Mississippi, Pokey and I resumed out normal routine of work and school, feeling that my return home was anticlimactic at best.

During the process, it is customary for annual conferences in the United Methodist Church to send teams to each of the theology schools where students from that conference attend to meet with students and their families. The process is billed as a "checking on you" visit, but the real purpose is to make sure that seminary students remain connected to their home conferences and plan to serve there in ministry. Several officials make the trip, usually meeting with the students at the seminary itself and following up with a meal at a local restaurant or church.

Our visit that January was scheduled for a local church outside Durham. When Pokey and I arrived at the meal, we met two district superintendents from Mississippi who had arrived to meet us and the other students. We briefly talked with both gentlemen and then spent the rest of the evening sitting at the end of the table talking with friends.

At the end of the meeting, Reverend Jones asked if he and Reverend Nicholson, the other superintendent, could get a ride back to their hotel, just a few miles away in Durham. This was out of our way, and other students lived closer, but Reverend Jones insisted that we take them home, so we all packed into Pokey's compact Mazda and drove off.

When we arrived at the hotel, Pokey and I began to feel nervous as Reverend Nicholson asked us to come inside to talk about my interview and the upcoming Board of Ministry meeting. The feeling intensified when he told us Larry Goodpaster was staying at the same hotel. We were escorted to Reverend Goodpaster's room. Pokey and I liked Larry very much. He was kind, soft spoken, and gracious. He was also apologetic for the secret maneuverings of the evening, but he didn't want the other students to know he was in town or to give any inkling as to the severity of my issue. The bishop and he had orchestrated this meeting, he told us, to discuss my ordination process and possible roadblocks.

Larry's demeanor immediately calmed us, and Pokey and I

sat on the sofa while the others sat in chairs and on the corner of the bed. The whole scene was straight out of a spy movie as we huddled to discuss our strategy for the ordination process.

"Well, I know this all seems strange and a little over the top, but the bishop and I believed we should have these conversations with you face-to-face," Larry said. "You know that your health is a delicate issue for our board and your appointability."

Appointability. That was the key issue for ordination. United Methodists have guaranteed appointments, meaning that once you are ordained, the church is responsible for finding you a job. But if I couldn't be appointed, could I be ordained? Larry worried that we might go through the ordination process without a hitch and still not be able to find a church that would take me as their pastor.

For the next two hours, we examined the process from every possible angle. We agreed we would move forward, although everyone in the room knew that we had two challenges: convincing the Board of Ordained Ministry that I could be ordained and appointed—then making the appointment work.

Reverend Jones noted that he had not seen a time in his ministry when the ethical, theological, spiritual, and practical issues of the church's life were more intersected, or when more was at stake in aligning them. We all knew that if just one of the questions could not be answered, the entire process was in jeopardy.

Before Pokey and I left the room, Larry put his arms around us and said a prayer for guidance, courage, and strength. We needed all of those in greater measure than we ever imagined, and it felt good to have someone pray for us.

When Pokey and I arrived home from the meeting, we were both in shock. We talked late into the evening. After Pokey fell asleep, I sat awake, trying to read my Bible. Even with the encouragement from Larry about the process and his and the bishop's resolve in the matter, I was frustrated and worried. All I wanted was to finish my training and pastor a local church. I had a disease that I was doing my best to live through, but maybe my disease, I realized for the first time, was bigger than me.

DELIBERATIONS

The Board of Ministry met in early spring. Nancy Tatum attended to answer medical questions. After much discussion, the debate finally landed at the issue of appointability. One person suggested that appointing me would be unfair both to me and to the church. What would happen if I were to be ordained and then no one would take me? How would that affect me, my family, or my health? Further, what about the congregation and their safety? Could they afford to appoint an HIV positive pastor to a church with the possibility that there could be an accident and someone could be infected? What about those who were too afraid to attend church because of my health condition? What about losing a pastor painfully and publicly?

These were legitimate questions with no easy answers. Though I could tell he took no pleasure in asking them, the man took us to the core of the matter. "Do we not have a responsibility to those people?" he asked.

As the meeting progressed, Rocky Miskelly, the young minister who had been advocating for me from the very beginning, asked a stunning question. "I have heard a lot of talk about whether we can afford to ordain this young man, about his health, the church, liability, insurance — you name it. But I would like to pose this question: Can we afford not to ordain him?"

The board went silent.

Rocky continued, "Can we afford to take a person whose theological work has been superb, as acknowledged by everyone here, and not ordain him based on his physical condition?"

Rocky continued, standing and turning to those in the back of the room. "Can we afford to take a person whose moral character has never been in question, and has, in fact, only been praised by those who have spoken on his behalf, and *not* ordain him based on a virus in his bloodstream?"

The room remained silent. Rocky turned this time to the group that had been the most vocal against ordination, sitting together on the other side of the room in the rear. "Can we afford to take a person who, according to the videotaped sermon we saw, possesses such strong gifts as a communicator and not ordain him because he lives, mind you, with a disease?"

Again, silence.

Rocky now turned back toward the podium and the bishop and chair. "But most importantly, I ask you, can we afford to take a person who is willing, himself, to face the prejudice and discrimination and struggles that this journey may bring him, and not ordain him because we are afraid of what that journey might mean to us or to our churches?"

"The real question, I believe," Rocky continued, "is that if we do not ordain him, can we afford ...?" He paused and looked down, then continued again. "No, let me ask it this way: Do we deserve to be called the body of Christ?"

The conversation from that point took a very different tone. Larry called for a vote, and the board overwhelmingly voted to

recommend ordination to the clergy session of the annual conference, which would meet in June. Larry, after the vote, called
everyone to a moment of silence and then offered a prayer about
courage and unity.

Although there were a few dissenters, the majority of my
brothers and sisters spoke into my life — and the life of our
church — with faith and hope. The Mississippi United Methodist Church had just become the first mainline denominational
body to ordain an openly HIV positive minister.

Of course, this was neither the end of the questions nor the
end of the road. The struggle had only begun. But the details of
objecting to my ordination now stood in contrast to the moral
imperative of the gospel and a qualified candidate for ministry. This candidate had a real name and real, committed people
speaking on his behalf and asking important questions about
the life of the church. The tide had turned, and issues like death
benefits and insurance, as important as they were, seemed less
important than following Christ's command to preach the gospel. Of course, not everyone was sold, and some continued to
oppose the ordination. But no matter how logical the argument,
it was hard to contend with the sentiments of the gospel imperative, especially since my calling had never been in question.

This venue served as a valuable lesson about this conversation in other settings. Not every place where the issue of ordaining me would be debated would have the bishop and a medical
adviser to respond. And given the complex nature of the issues,
it would take a great deal of patience.

The people who most impacted the issue were those in the
pews who had to balance their good, Christian notions of right
and wrong with the fear and knowledge of HIV/AIDS. And no

matter how many boards or committees to whom we made our case, the regular members in the pews were the ones who made the final call. What remained was to convince laypersons of the same information and insight we had provided for the committee members and then to find a pulpit I could call home.

Chapter 6

CONVERSATIONS FOR OTHER PLACES

We leave North Carolina today. I will drive back with Patty (my mother-in-law) and Pokey, and Nanny will come in the next few days. Just two years ago we were petrified about being here by ourselves. Now we feel like we are leaving family. Funny how God brings people together when we let him.

—Journal entry, June 1994

As the ordination process had increased in complexity, Pokey and I had shared with more and more people at Benson Memorial about my health. At first it was more of a response from our Sunday school class, since they could sense the stress we were under most. Next, we shared the information with the church's staff parish relations committee (the personnel committee) followed by the general board. We discovered that the congregation was very open (especially after we learned the tremendous legwork the class had put into talking with others about the issue). They had contacted nearly every council member and had with one large stroke alleviated many of the people's fears. We also had built a significant amount of community and inroads in the congregation *before* the information came out. They already knew us, which, as we would learn time and again, made a tremendous difference.

Benson Memorial asked me to remain on staff after completing theology school. Our intention had always been to return to Mississippi, but the offer from Benson Memorial was certainly enticing. It was also important, because they were answering the appointability question for the ordination process. Here was a church that wanted me and had no problem with my disease. I had loved serving at Benson, getting to know people, but most important in this issue, they had come to know me. I would never underestimate the importance of knowing and being known again.

During this time, I received other offers for positions as well. One in particular was very intriguing. Larry Goodpaster, the chair of the Mississippi Board of Ordained Ministry, and one of the men who had met us in the clandestine hotel meeting months earlier, called to inquire about our interest in serving on staff with him at a large, growing congregation in Mississippi. The thought of working with Larry was attractive, not to mention affirming. Larry, who would later be elected bishop in the United Methodist Church, was well respected, and working with him added another layer of credibility to my ordination. It also provided some security in what had grown into an unsettling process, to say the least.

However, in the spring, Pokey's grandfather passed away unexpectedly. After the funeral, and while we were still in Mississippi, the district superintendent informed us that an appointment as a pastor to a small church just twenty miles north of Hattiesburg had become a possibility, and he wanted to know if we were interested. With our concern for family members following her grandfather's death, we felt an appointment closer to home would be best and thus graciously declined the offers from Benson Memorial and from Larry.

The appointment was approved. However, the local superintendent, in all of his conversations with the local church in question, had not mentioned any of my health issues. Looking back, it seems odd that he would not have done so, but he believed that this was information that needed to be shared in person by me. I understand his thinking, but it may have saved a lot of heartache to have broached the issue earlier.

In the United Methodist Church, when a new pastor is appointed, a covenant meeting is scheduled between the new pastor and the church in order for both parties to meet, ask questions, and get to know one another better. It was also a time to talk through various issues that might affect the appointment. Unlike in some denominations, it is not a time for any voting for approval. That responsibility in the UMC is given to the bishop and the cabinet, an annual conference's district superintendents and assistants to the bishop, alone.

By late April my covenant meeting had been scheduled, and I made plans to drive the fourteen hours to Mississippi and meet my new parishioners. A friend, who was also in theology school and from Mississippi, rode with me.

While we were driving down to Mississippi, Pokey received a message at work saying that the district superintendent from Mississippi was trying to get in touch with me. This was certainly odd, but Pokey thought it had something to do with the meeting scheduled for the next evening. When she returned his call, the superintendent told Pokey that the night before, the church had called a special meeting to consider new information about me. Someone in the congregation had heard about my health and was, naturally, concerned about my appointment as pastor. "During the meeting," the superintendent said, "the congregation voted — though they technically did not have this right — to veto Shane as their pastor."

"What does this mean? How difficult is the situation? I mean, are they really panicked or just concerned?" Pokey asked.

"Some have said that they will not allow him to baptize their children, and ..."

There was a long pause on the other end.

"And *what*?" Pokey prompted.

"Someone threatened to burn down the parsonage if you move in," the superintendent answered.

I remember the drive well, because my friend and I were stopped for speeding in Jefferson County, Georgia. I had just started taking a new, experimental medicine that came in white tablets and had to be pulverized into powder and mixed with water before I could take it. Pokey, who was always trying to organize my meds better and make sure I took them accurately, had taken several pulverized doses and placed each of them in clear ziplock bags. Imagine the scene: The officer pulls us over and sees a row of bags filled with white powder in the backseat. I tried to explain what the medicine was for, going into long detail about my condition. I am not sure if he really believed me or if he just let us go because it was the best excuse he had ever heard. Regardless, we were given a speeding ticket and were on our way.

When I arrived at my mother's house later that evening, I could tell almost immediately that something wasn't right. Normally she was very affectionate and jealous of my attention, but from the moment my feet hit the ground, she insisted that I call Pokey at home. I kept trying to put her off, until finally she said, "Shane, Pokey needs to tell you something."

I dialed our number, suddenly nervous.

"Sweetheart," Pokey said, "the church had a meeting last night and voted not to take you as their pastor."

I made her repeat what she had said.

"But they can't vote!"

"Well, they think they can," Pokey replied. "And they did. The superintendent called me earlier today."

We talked for several minutes about the other parts of the superintendent's conversation. He wanted me to visit the bishop the next day and make plans for how to proceed from here. We had been prepared for resistance, but people had always come around—even the tough ones—when they got to know us. Our hope was that once a church knew us, they would feel better about my health situation. What we hadn't considered is what would happen when people heard about me before meeting me. Most people who have concerns about my health raise valid issues from a sense of genuine inquiry. This congregation, however, had responded out of something more insidious—fear.

Pokey and I finished the call by praying for one another. It was a tough moment, and both of us could tell the other was having trouble praying. We weren't frustrated with God but with the church. God's people have a way of making things complicated and creating many of their own troubles.

Before I hung up the phone, I asked Pokey, "You still okay about doing this?"

"Doing what?" she asked.

"You, me, and this crazy journey," I replied, half joking but also wondering how much this young, beautiful woman would want to take.

"More than ever," she said. "More than ever."

We expressed our love for each other and hung up. I would realize later that my question to Pokey was more for me than her. I loved her with all of my heart, but I was all the more determined not to allow these situations to define us. Something started happening within me that night that would take years for me to admit. I set myself up against the expectations and prejudices of others, and I was determined that nothing—nothing—would keep me from accomplishing my goals and proving my detractors wrong. There was something even darker, as well: a desire to make them regret that they had not taken a chance on me. What I couldn't know or understand at the time was that in taking on that attitude, I took a bit of myself back from God. It was becoming about me, rather than God and his church, and in trying to be strong, I opened up a chink in my own armor through which I would be wounded later.

The next day I met with the bishop who, throughout the process, had been a fierce supporter. It was not hard to read his heart or to hear the commitment in his voice. However, our conversation went differently than I expected. I assumed that he would simply make another appointment, but he requested that I attend the covenant meeting at the church as planned.

I was stunned. I had no intention of attending. Seeing my confusion, the bishop assured me he had no intention of appointing me to this congregation, but he wanted to send a signal that this process is not about human conditions or perceptions but about faithfulness and doing the right thing.

He also wanted me to attend the meeting because he believed these people needed to take responsibility for their choice. "The church's board has overstepped its authority," he said. "For them to make this decision and not have any accountability would be a far greater mistake than even what they are doing and thinking now. The church is walking a dangerous, fine line spiritually in deciding for themselves who can be part of the family and who cannot."

I hadn't thought of it in those terms before. This had been about me, the church, and the office of pastor, but there was a wider issue. If a local church could do this to me, then what signal would their concerns send to anyone attending their fellowship or the church at large?

"The doors of the church are always open no matter what our fears may be," the bishop said.

For several minutes the bishop and I sat quietly in his office. I don't think either of us could really believe that we were confronting this issue.

"I need you to go for them, Shane," the bishop finally said.

There are moments in biblical story when people—for instance, Abraham, Isaiah, Jonah, and Paul—are called to go to difficult places they know will, in some ways, break them. We may know missionaries or social workers who go to such places every day, but few of us experience the dilemma of being called "to go" in the midst of real crisis and danger.

I understood the bishop's request, even with my reservations, and understood that sitting across the table from people who feared me, or maybe even despised me, was at the heart of the gospel—the real gospel. Such moments shape the body of Christ and make us ready to do what we are created to do.

The next night the superintendent and I arrived for the covenant meeting. The more vocal church members who opposed my appointment did not show up. The ones who came looked as though someone had drained the spirit from them. Their sadness and regret were palpable, written in their downcast eyes and their twisting, nervous hands. It took only a few minutes for me to realize that the Lord placed me there to minister to them in their grief, not the other way around. I spent the better part of the meeting listening to their fears, prayers, and confessions. It was a tough meeting, but one also filled with grace and forgiveness.

As I left, I looked across the churchyard to the parsonage. Pokey and I had driven by the house while we were in Hattiesburg, months earlier, for her grandfather's funeral. Thinking we were going to live in that house, we had talked for several weeks about what our new life would be like. Now it stood silent and empty in the darkness. But at least it stood unburned, waiting for a minister who would come to help this congregation heal and, by God's grace, grow.

HERITAGE

For a person who believes he or she is called to ministry and who spends the time to prepare and train for that calling, being rejected by a local church feels like being kicked in the stomach. Eventually I would get my breath back, but I was different. My love for God had not changed, but my trust of God's people certainly had. It would take several years before I regained much of my passion and outlook for the church. I was also different in that I felt that my ministry was placed under a microscope. If I were to succeed, I would need to give more than others and then make sure that people knew about it. I wanted people to feel good about their "investment," but more than anything, to simply like me. I couldn't stay bent over forever — I had to get up and move on. But I always remembered being kicked, and somewhere deep inside I was watching for the next blow.

Two days after the covenant meeting, I received a call from the pastor of Heritage UMC in Hattiesburg, our hometown. Heritage was the new name for the church Pokey had grown up in and that I had joined when I became a Methodist. Heritage had relocated from its original location to a fast-growing side of the city, and now it needed an associate pastor. Heavy debt loads from construction projects had prevented the congregation from affording an associate pastor full-time. The pastor learned of my situation and shared the scenario with several people in the congregation. Many of the members had prayed for Pokey and me over the years and were, of course, heartbroken at our recent circumstances.

One person saw these circumstances as an opportunity and a moving of God's hand for both us and for her church. Ms. Polly was a surrogate mother to everyone. When I was in college, I could show up at her house for tomato sandwiches anytime—a delicacy for a starving student. Ms. Polly loved her church and in recent months realized the need for another minister to help with the growing congregation. A day after my covenant meeting with the other church, she walked into the pastor's office at Heritage and wrote a check that was the equivalent of two years' salary for an associate pastor. Ms. Polly asked that it be used to fund a position at the church for me. The pastor contacted the bishop, who contacted me and shared the news.

Still, Pokey and I were cautious. We had learned to rely on each other, and accepting this offer at first felt like giving in to our fears and doing the easy thing. Yet we could not overlook the unbelievable grace of this gift, and we had to admit that safety and security in a place we knew sounded wonderful.

That didn't mean that everyone at Heritage knew of and accepted my health condition. I hadn't talked openly about it when I served part-time on staff. The pastor had to do his own groundwork for this new position, including confronting the issue of my health for those at Heritage who might have questions. After a lengthy and honest discussion, the administrative board of the church voted to confirm my new position by a count of 48 to 0, with 1 abstention. I learned later that the lone abstaining voter turned out to be one of my greatest supporters during my time at the church.

During the next weeks, Pokey and I returned to North Carolina, and I finished my theology degree at Duke while Pokey finished her master's degree at Meredith College. With everything else going on, we still had the normal requirements for graduation as the other students. It was a busy, stressful time. Most important, Pokey and I said good-bye to our friends and church family in North Carolina, a tough, bittersweet time. We moved back to Hattiesburg and rented a house not far from the church.

During the summer, Pokey and I settled into our new home and our new church. She found a job teaching at the local elementary school, and I jumped headlong into my role as associate pastor at Heritage UMC. It felt good to put the stress of our recent past behind us although—and we didn't know it at the time—we were creating a system for other stresses.

Deep down, however, and little realized by either of us, the rejection of that first appointment had profoundly affected us. Pokey was made wary and bitter; she became suspicious of people's motives. What were people *really* thinking about us? Even though the folks at Heritage had accepted us, did they really understand and accept us completely? I became driven to prove to everyone that I was worth their risk—to be so dedicated and productive in my job as to be the best at what I did. In my mind, it wasn't enough to be good; I had to be exceptional. That meant long hours at the church. This was our first experience of confronting the burden of carrying my condition in the context of a public pastorate. The pressures and assessments we put on ourselves and believed others were adding, as they continued to mount, would eventually be too much to bear.

Pokey faced difficult emotional transitions too. Perhaps for the first time, she saw how vulnerable my condition made us and how it pushed me to work too hard, even at the expense of our relationship. Moving back to the safety of her family provided a short-term fix for those fears, but it also stole a piece of the independence that Pokey had discovered living on her own. That independence had provided an important context for us as a couple. It made us rely on each other first instead of running to family. During our time in North Carolina, we had learned to work out our differences, fears, and hopes together. Moving home changed that.

We were more wounded than we admitted, but we muddled through without making much of a fuss or discussing our feelings in depth, either with each other or with our friends. Responding to the need to both prove ourselves and somehow dull the sting of what we had faced, we began to speed through life—sometimes inadvertently leaving each other behind. It is important to understand that just months or years earlier, such treatment of each other would have been unthinkable. We had always been best friends and each other's number one advocate. But the stress of the past months had served to create dynamics in each of us that we had never seen before. And worse yet, it all unfolded in ways that were not easily recognizable until we were way down an unhealthy road. For instance, Pokey and I always went everywhere together or were always careful not to be in situations that might look inappropriate. However, within a few months of moving home, I was busy with friends and members of the church, often going out to eat without Pokey or spending time with friends on the weekends without Pokey. Nothing inappropriate happened, but it sent a signal to her and others of our priorities. Pokey, on the other hand, began spending a lot of time volunteering for events at school and, since she was working in a special class setting that would eventually be her research project, spending a lot of time going to sporting and special events of her students. During this time, a strong friendship with another man ensued, and, again, though nothing inappropriate happened during this time, it provided for a relationship that otherwise would not have been expected or tolerated in our marriage. In fact, the more time I spent working and being involved with the church, the more I left Pokey open to this other relationship.

Pokey and I were not oblivious to the temptations and struggles in our marriage. Just after arriving at Heritage for our new appointment, we attended a marriage retreat weekend. Pokey and I talked a lot about what we were feeling and about how we knew that life no longer felt like it used to. The conversation bothered us so much that we sought help from the retreat leader, who provided some great insight about ways that we could stay connected and about the importance of making each other first no matter what came our way. It was especially important, he reiterated, that we rely on and support each other. The danger to our marriage, he warned, was not so much complete destruction as it was gradual erosion and distraction.

We recognized the warning signs. In struggling to keep the disease from defining us in one way, we were allowing it to define us in another way by driving us to move through life too quickly. The marriage retreat meant a lot to us. Pokey and I both kept journals of our time together, and we were both willing to listen to what the retreat leader was saying. However, as soon as we returned home, the forces pulling at us did not let up, and within no time, we were back to old patterns. Pokey and I both were ready to make things work; we clearly loved each other. But unfortunately, as we learned later in our marriage, even in one as close as ours, love is not enough, and we couldn't see the wreck coming just around the corner.

THE WRECK

Just a few months into our time at Heritage, the senior pastor was involved in a serious car accident. Though he did not have any life-threatening injuries, the accident left him in the hospital for several weeks and recovering at home for many more.

During his absence, I assumed the duties of pastor for the congregation. It was an intense time. We had just entered a new visioning campaign that resulted in the creation of multiple worship services and several staff realignments. With the pastor injured, I was left to handle these changes. Of course, I was also dealing with my own internal struggles, and everything in life became a race of sorts, including my relationship with the church and with God.

I again began working extremely long hours at the church and spending even less time with Pokey. Neither of us had experienced this before. Pokey's response was to focus on her classroom, enmesh herself in old, unhealthy family relationships, and spend more time in this new friend relationship that was clearly headed in a dangerous direction. Everything in our marriage changed so quickly that within eighteen months, Pokey and I had grown apart in ways that only two years before would have seemed impossible. I couldn't (or wouldn't) explain my new-found sense of rushing obligation; Pokey couldn't (or wouldn't) express her loneliness and growing bitterness toward so many aspects of our life together.

Ironically, we were both excelling in our professional lives.

From the outside, we looked like a successful couple. Our personal life, however, was growing more fractured, and worst of all, neither of us could explain it to the other. That would require opening up very fragile places in our lives that neither of us was prepared to confront. Instead, we simply trudged further into danger.

Most people who knew us assumed that our journey gave us some relational superstructure to protect us from such attacks. But we were prone to the same relational stresses and complexities as other couples. We had been through much together, but like any married couple, as our focus left each other, our relationship began to experience serious cracks that spread like spiderwebs into every corner of our lives. Pokey became emotionally intimate with another man; the other woman in my life was the church. Each of us felt enormous guilt, and a determination — born of love — to make our marriage work. But we needed to be on the same team, working together. Instead, whether from pride or fear, we were working in isolation from each other. A married couple, we were living alone, together.

In North Carolina we couldn't wait to come home and cook dinner together. We enjoyed eating in front of the television, enjoying one of our favorite shows. However, over the previous months, we would come home from work to separate meals or leftovers, often eating in different rooms. One evening I came home to experience another long, quiet night of distance between the two of us, when I realized that Pokey had already gone to take a bath and get ready for bed. I walked into the bathroom to find Pokey lying in a tub of warm water staring aimlessly into space.

"What are you thinking about?" I asked.

Finally, after several seconds, Pokey looked up with tears in her eyes. "Let's just pack up and go back to North Carolina."

I couldn't believe her words. She continued: "We can get jobs somewhere. I'll teach; Benson Memorial will hire you back...." Her sobs became more apparent, more worried. She got out of the tub and walked over to me, dripping and naked. She put her arms around me and continued to speak, even as the warm water soaked into my clothes. "We can get our old apartment back and get back to living life like it used to be. Please tell me we can do that.... I don't care what happens to our house or our jobs here.... Just please, please, let's get out of here."

By this time she was weeping. I picked her up and laid her on our bed. She was shivering, balled up in a fetal position. I placed a blanket on her and lay down beside her. I put my arms around her, and we slept there the entire night.

In the morning, she woke up, got dressed, and left for work.

Looking back, I wish we had packed our clothes and headed out of town that night. But we didn't. I couldn't. There was too much to do and take care of and watch out for. I went back to my life at the church, responsible as always to take care of the flock and make sure that everyone in my life was taken care of, with the exception of the one person who mattered most. Pokey went back to her classroom and began work on her doctorate, taking the prescribed classes before residency would be required. During this time, she also allowed her friendship with this other person to go out of control, and Pokey believed that, during this time, she fell in love with him. Now, not only had I lost the time and opportunity to make things right with her, but I had lost part of her heart as well. Of course, I didn't realize the full nature of what was happening. On the surface, Pokey and I remained as strong as ever. And to her credit, she kept showing up at all of the church events and playing the part of the good pastor's wife. All the while, though, she had found her escape and would spend more and more time in that place. Yes, I most certainly wished we had packed up and moved away. Several years would pass before Pokey's silence broke again, and by that time, I would nearly lose her for good.

HELLOS

Pokey and I believed we would never be able to have children. We had planned our lives without the possibility of ever being parents. Both of us seemed satisfied with this until a friend of ours told us of a procedure whereby Pokey and the baby would be safe from contracting HIV and, if a girl, from even becoming a carrier of hemophilia. Pokey was excited. I, however, was still skeptical, not because I didn't want to have a family with Pokey, but because so much of the future was uncertain. I was afraid of my health failing and Pokey being left as a young widow — the thought of her being a young widow and a young mom was all the more difficult.

We were also worried about how we would explain our decision to others. Having a child would only increase the questions and scrutiny. Adoption was prohibitively difficult because of my HIV status. If we were to have a family, the procedure suggested by our friend was our only hope, especially in terms of the long-term health of everyone involved.

Pokey and I loved children, and we concluded that, regardless of how much time I had or what people thought or how complicated it might be, we wanted to share that love with a child of our own. We had spent a lot of time over the past months working apart from one another instead of in the same direction. We believed a baby would certainly help us rediscover our relationship, and so we made our first appointment with the doctor to try the new procedure.

Trying to get pregnant was not the only new beginning we were planning. A month earlier, the district superintendent asked me to consider planting a new church in Petal, a community just to the east of Hattiesburg. Petal, as you might recall, was the small town where Nancy's medical clinic was located. At first I declined, wanting to stay at Heritage, especially as Pokey and I were planning to start a family. But the Lord had other plans. Members from a core group of laypeople who had committed to start the new congregation had been visiting Heritage through-out the late fall and winter and had heard me preach on several occasions. I learned later they had shamelessly lobbied the super-intendent to name me as the new pastor. The superintendent finally convinced me to meet with the core group about their ideas. I reluctantly agreed, thinking that such a meeting would finally put the discussion to rest.

Pokey and I attended the meeting, and by the end, I was hooked. The group was small but genuine, and they had cer-tainly "prayed up," as my grandmother would say. They answered every question I asked, including whether they thought the com-munity would be okay with my HIV status. I would no longer entertain an appointment as pastor unless I could be straightfor-ward about my health. No one in the core group objected. Sev-eral said my transparency was one of the reasons they believed God had led them to me.

As we discussed how people might feel about joining a new

church and learning that their pastor was HIV positive, I noticed a big, tough-looking guy at the end of the table struggling to stand. Lonny was a football coach at the local high school. He looked every bit the part, standing well over six feet tall with broad shoulders and huge hands. But as he stood, I noticed something unusual about him. He steadied himself with his hands, and then like a robot in an old sci-fi movie, turned to face me. As I looked closer, I could tell that Lonny wore prosthetic legs from the knees down. Lonny had been hit by a drunk driver while a freshman in college. The girl he was walking home that evening was killed instantly. Lonny lost the bottom of both legs.

As Lonny turned toward me in the meeting, I remember seeing tears in his eyes, and then he spoke: "I think we would be honored to have you as our pastor, not in spite of your disease, but because of it. I don't want my children to think the world is a scary place, but I also don't want them to think it is perfect either. What I want more than anything is for them to see that in spite of the imperfections, we have a choice to overcome our struggles and make something of our lives," he continued. "I know as well as anyone that we are all broken somewhere. Let's take whatever any of us have, good or bad, and go forward in this." The rest of the group gave a resounding "Amen!"

Lonny's words reminded me that what we do on this earth is best done together, and over the years, it would be a joy to work side by side with Lonny as we built the church, from laying sod outside the new building to holding the hands of those taking their final breaths. Over our ministry together, Lonny became more than my parishioner — he became my example and friend.

As the meeting came to a close, Pokey received a call on her cell phone from the doctor's office informing us that she was pregnant. She turned to me and said, "It's positive." That was the first time I had heard those words in such a happy way. Two years earlier, neither Pokey nor I could have imagined such a gift. She touched my hand and looked me in the eyes. Even for that short moment, we felt the connection again between us and knew that, in spite of so many difficult moments, what we had was worth fighting for.

It was a night of new beginnings: a new church and a new baby.

Chapter 7

THE COST OF WHAT
WE CANNOT AFFORD

*A minister friend came today to visit me, but I was hurting
so bad I couldn't even keep my eyes open. But today was
also very special. I was ordained tonight, ushered from my
hospital bed through a back door onto a stage. It's funny if
you think about it. The needle still in my arm, but looking
dapper in my robe. Patty and I got some ice cream when I
got back to the hospital. My fever came back. I threw up the
ice cream. Well. Such is life.*

—Journal entry, June 1996

My great-aunt liked to say, "It won't take many steps before you discover whether Satan is happy about the path you have chosen." I always thought it odd that she didn't reference God in this saying, but her point was that God goes with you even when you take a difficult or a wrong turn. Satan, on the other hand, when he sees you take a path that leads to something good for the kingdom, stops at nothing to disqualify, frustrate, or discomfort the journey.

The decision to start a new church must have scared Satan silly, because from the beginning we were faced with one obstacle after the other. Within the first weeks of accepting the appointment, I suffered a severe reaction to new medicines used to treat my HIV. High fevers and rashes were draining and painful. Just a week before I was supposed to be ordained as an elder (the final ordination in the process for United Methodists), I was hospitalized for a high fever and a high blood sugar count. Doctors advised me not to attend the ordination, but after having put so much work into the process and not wanting to let anyone have the "I told you so" moment, I convinced them to let me check out of the hospital and attend. The annual conference met in Jackson, and since it was June, the heat was unbelievable. Pokey, by this time, was also feeling the full effects of morning sickness.

After just one day of attending the conference, my fever returned, and I found myself admitted to the hospital in Jackson. Since Nancy lived and worked in Jackson, she could oversee my care personally. But I was missing one of the most important times of my professional career, and the thought of not attending my ordination was troubling. Because the fevers came on frequently and it would take nearly three weeks to get the medicines to which I reacted out of my system completely, sitting through the services was not an option, and I was advised to consider my health and not attend.

Rocky Miskelly, the young minister who had defended me at the first Board of Ministry meeting and who had become a dear friend, developed a plan whereby I could leave the hospital, be transported to the convention center where the conference and worship service were being held, be ordained, and then be returned to the hospital that evening. The key was to time the fever spike at just the right moment with medicine so that I would feel good enough to make the transition. The bishop and Nancy approved the plan, and Rocky, along with several other members of the board, made arrangements.

But first I had to receive the "Questions for Ministry," a process that normally took place in front of the entire conference. The bishop sent his administrative assistant to administer the "Questions" in my hospital room an hour or so before the service. When the service began, Rocky called my mother-in-law, Patty, who had volunteered to be the driver in our plan, and told her it was time. Other family members, including Pokey, sat waiting in the family section at the convention center. Dressed in my suit, and with my robe in hand, we drove to the convention center, complete with the IV (capped and filled with heparin to keep it from clotting) still in my arm.

We arrived at the back door loading dock of the convention center, and I was escorted around the curtains to the end of the stage. Usually candidates are ordained in alphabetical order, but I was placed at the front of the line.

When it came time for me to kneel at the altar and be ordained, the bishop, along with other elders that I had asked to be a part of the ceremony, placed his hands on my head. He paused a minute and looked over me and noticed the crowd. It is common at our ordinations for friends and relatives to stand as their loved one is being ordained. When the bishop saw the crowd, he gave an audible gasp. He then smiled and whispered into my ear, "Shane, they are all standing for you."

Tears filled my eyes. What had begun so many years ago, with all of the roadblocks and questions, had come full circle, and many who had once refused to look me in the eye now stood in support. The bishop, tears in his own eyes, regained his composure and began the ordination, He placed his hands on my head and repeated the ordination ritual: "Almighty God, pour upon Larry Shane Stanford the Holy Spirit, for the office and work of an elder. Amen. Larry Shane Stanford, take authority as an elder in the Church to preach the Word of God, and to administer the Holy Sacraments in the name of the Father, and the Son, and the Holy Spirit. Amen."

When the bishop was finished speaking, the congregation answered with their own "Amen."

I was able to return to Hattiesburg a week later. I was still very weak from the fevers but was excited about starting my new job. Pastoral appointment changes happen within the two- to three-week period following the annual conference. I was scheduled to preach my first sermon at the new church in Petal, which was waiting on me before selecting a name. When I arrived at the Petal Community Center, I still had a Hep-loc (a portable

IV) in my arm. To make matters worse, a few days after I arrived home, I developed another rash in response to the antibiotics I was given in the hospital. I was quite a sight: the new preacher arriving with gadgets sticking out of his arm and what looked like a world-class sunburn. It is a wonder the people of that new church didn't ask for a reconsideration.

In fact, they went out of their way to make me feel comfortable. They were patient, caring, and understanding, and I knew that I had made the right decision in accepting this appointment.

What no one knew was the struggle Pokey and I were enduring at the same time. The night after my head-to-toe rash broke out, Pokey took me to the doctor to get a shot for the extreme itching and discomfort. The doctor who gave the shot failed to note that I was a hemophiliac and gave me the injection in a muscle using a needle that caused a lot of tissue damage. This, in turn, started a bleed in a muscle near my hip, which by the next day had turned into full-blown internal hemorrhage. I would need several doses of Factor VIII to make the bleeding stop. Nancy prescribed the Factor to be given every eight hours for a week. Pokey, who had been trained years before, was used to giving the medicines to me at home.

One of the doses on the schedule had to be administered at midnight. Two nights into the dosage schedule, Pokey mixed the medicine and gave me the shot as I slept on the sofa, which was the most comfortable place for me to rest. I woke up just as she finished pushing the last drop of Factor through the needle. When she turned to leave and discard the needle, her foot caught on the edge of the coffee table and she tripped.

The needle broke the skin of her left hand.

Pokey jerked out the needle and went quickly to the sink.

Since I wasn't moving well, it took me a minute to get up. By the time I got to Pokey, her eyes were filled with tears, and so were mine. We had feared this happening, and now—despite our best efforts at caution—it had.

Pokey was four months pregnant.

That week was one of the worst of our lives. Pokey's HIV test, at last, came back negative, and all subsequent tests, including those taken just after the baby was born, revealed nothing. It would not be the last such test we would endure. There is a particular helpless agony in waiting for the results of blood tests that will, in a single moment, change your life. Just after the negative results of Pokey's tests came in, we learned that my immune system had continued to deteriorate and now only responded at about 3 percent of normal.

What could we do? Our life together had become a series of tests, one after another—a series of numbers, reports, and phone calls. Looking back, we should have slowed down. But as before, we kept pushing forward.

Survival isn't always about heroics; often it's a matter of simply standing. I love Paul's phrase from Ephesians 6 where he is talking about the armor of God: "after you have done all you can do to stand . . . then stand" (v. 13, my paraphrase). It seems anticlimactic, but when you have been in the middle of a storm, you know exactly what he is talking about. In any storm—physical, emotional, spiritual, financial—standing is not a given. Standing says we are here to fight and not give in.

When we stand, we do more than announce our determination to survive. We declare that we never stand alone, for no storm can drive us from the side of our ever-faithful God.

THE IMPORTANCE OF PLACE

When we stand, we always stand in a place. As broken people, we need something foundational upon which we can build our lives and hopes. This isn't only a physical place, but something deeper, and it is one of the hardest things for those of us struggling with the displacement of chronic illness to discover.

We long to sense that we belong to something or someone that the world cannot change. I believe it is the archetypical ache Adam and Eve felt when they were forced to leave the garden, and each person has felt that same ache in myriad ways ever since.

I learned this firsthand from a friend named Tommy who literally arrived on our doorstep while we were still serving at Heritage. He was thin, sickly, and obviously in distress. Tommy was crushed by regret and the consequences of bad decisions. That day he found himself standing on the doorstep of a stranger, a preacher, desperate to believe in anything. *Anything.*

Tommy and I didn't have much in common beyond our common diagnoses of HIV. He was tall, opinionated, and flamboyant. I was more reserved and reflective. But over the year-and-a-half that we met together to talk about life, we discovered another bond: Our grandmothers had both loved to sing "Jesus Loves Me" to us. Tommy's grandmother had passed away many years earlier, but he could still remember the sound of her voice and the way it gave him a sense of belonging.

Tommy became active on our church's music team. One day I received a call; Tommy was in the hospital. By the time I arrived, he was in and out of consciousness. When he realized where he was, he was unsettled and obviously distraught — his eyes were those of a man who would have taken off running as though something or someone was chasing him.

Nothing calmed him down. Everyone else had left his room, and I stood alone at the foot of his bed, thinking about the pain he felt and the fear flooding over him in that moment. This was not just about his physical body, but about his fear of what came next.

I took the blanket and pulled the covers up around his wasted body. As my grandmother did for me when I was a child, I tucked the blankets around Tommy and made sure that he was warm and snug. Then, like his grandmother, I leaned so close to him that our cheeks were touching, and I began to sing:

> *Jesus loves me this I know,*
> *For the Bible tells me so.*

He instantly calmed. I felt his body relax, and his eyes, so close to mine, closed. I continued to sing.

> *Little ones to him belong.*
> *They are weak, but he is strong.*
> *Yes, Jesus loves me.*
> *Yes, Jesus loves me.*
> *Yes, Jesus loves me.*
> *The Bible tells me so.*

The room was silent. By God's grace I had brought him to somewhere he could stand as the waters rose around him. The simple song reminded him of the simple story he believed, and about what was coming.

Tommy died the next day, asleep in his hospital bed but standing in his place.

NAMES

My mother named me after the movie *Shane* because she had a crush on Alan Ladd, the Western's straight-shooting star. *Shane* tells the story of a drifter who shows up in a frontier town looking for a new beginning, only to find himself engulfed in a battle with the local villain, played masterfully by Jack Palance. At the end of the movie, as Shane confronts Jack Wilson in the final showdown, he turns to Joey, the young boy who idolizes the gunslinger, and says, "You go home to your mother and father and grow up to be strong and straight." For Mom, the name Shane carried the idea of one who does the right thing and encourages others to do the same as well.

No pressure, right, Mom?

As Pokey and I moved to Petal and settled into our new role as church planters, we also prepared for life with a new baby. Pokey and I had thought about names for our new baby almost from the time we decided to get pregnant. We made a long list of possibilities but kept returning to one name in particular that had a significant meaning for us. A friend of ours had named her daughter Sarai the year before. This is the Hebrew spelling of Sarah and is the first name given to Abram's wife. It means "troublesome and quarrelsome," but it also symbolized what Sarai felt in not having children and in not feeling complete before giving birth to Isaac. It was only by grace from God that Sarai and Abraham were blessed with a child, and their lives — as well as all of history — would change forever.

Pokey and I, after finding out that we were definitely having a little girl, decided to name her Sarai Grace, after God's grace in giving us this wonderful, undeserved gift. In all honesty, we would not give as much theological consideration later to the names of our other two children, but Sarai Grace marked a new moment in our marriage and our relationship with God.

At the same time, we were also deciding on names for our new congregation. The congregational poll at the time had settled on "Grace" as the name of choice. I loved the name, having just decided to use it for our own daughter, but I wasn't totally convinced. I was reading a biography of Francis Asbury, founder of the Methodist Church in America. Asbury was a tenacious, faithful, somewhat disruptive figure who loved God and loved God's people. When the American War of Independence broke out, Asbury was the only Methodist preacher to remain in the Colonies, thus solidifying his reputation as a fierce example of justice and courage. Methodists, who had been tagged as Tories because of Wesley's support of the king, were being run out of the Colonies. Asbury refused to leave, thus securing the Methodist movement's future in America.

What a great example for our new congregation, I thought, *which has faced odds that other congregations would not have considered.* The day we chose the new name for the congregation, I launched into a detailed description of why I believed Asbury should be our name. Power to the pulpit, I say!

On September 8, 1996, Asbury United Methodist Church was officially chartered. In the founding documents of incorporation, we listed our motto as "A place of faith, family, and fellowship." Asbury was a remarkable new chapter that would forever change our lives. Later in the evening, the night of the official charter service, I wrote in my journal: "I cannot imagine a happier day in my professional life. I know that there will be other 'firsts' and other accomplishments, but how many pastors get to be at the start of something like this, and especially, with people like these?"

Like her namesake, Asbury Church was faithful, tenacious, and profound in the way it lived out its love for God. This congregation would, over our nearly ten years together, lead our community closer to the heart of God. More than anything, this congregation represented the possibilities we find when the body of Christ works together and trusts that what we do makes a difference. The odds this congregation and new pastor overcame testify to the wonderful grace of a God who knows us long before we know our own name.

HOPE IN SMALL HANDS

Sarai Grace Stanford was born on Friday, January 3, 1997. She was perfect from the beginning. After the nurses had given her a checkup, they handed her to me. She seemed so small and beautiful, almost like a doll. She was skinny with a wonderful glob of black hair on her head, and even from those first moments, she projected an air of sweet calm, a spirit she has kept to this day. I walked over to Pokey with the baby in my arms and leaned down and handed Sarai Grace to her mom. Our eyes were filled with tears as so many emotions ran through both of us. In our arms rested the blessing of so many struggles, sleepless nights, and uncertain tomorrows. Our lives would never be the same, we knew—and as so many friends with children had warned us!—and to reach this place with this new, perfect little being seemed like a miracle.

With Pokey holding the baby, we invited our family and friends into the room to share a prayer. My sister, Whitney, prayed a beautiful prayer, and we all cried and cheered together. As we adjusted to life with a new baby, Pokey and I felt like zombies, but happy ones nevertheless! We laughed and cried for no reason. As we welcomed this wonderful new gift into our lives, all of the stress and strain of the previous years seemed so far away.

Within a matter of weeks, Pokey and I resumed our normal duties, albeit with less sleep and more coffee. Pokey returned to the classroom, and I began work again at Asbury. That summer I received an invitation to speak at a student ministry conference in North Carolina and to share my story as an HIV positive minister. It was the first time I had been asked to share my story outside of Mississippi.

Other invitations quickly followed, and I found myself traveling more, sharing my testimony with churches, youth groups, and civic organizations. Later that year, the *Clarion Ledger*, Mississippi's largest newspaper, ran a front-page article about our family. According to Nancy, I was the poster boy for the new face of HIV, but I just felt like a juggler with too many balls in the air.

By this time, we had found a medicine cocktail that seemed to work, although the side effects were pretty tough, including fatigue, diarrhea, and various other periodic nuisances like thrush. The meds also changed the way I looked. My skin became dry and flaky with red splotches, and my body fat shifted positions. This was one of the more interesting, and disturbing, side effects. The medicines caused the fat tissue to move from my extremities to the center part of my body. One friend described me as looking like a rotten pear with toothpick limbs. What would I do without friends?

But the medicines worked, and that was the most important issue. Over the years, no matter how bad I felt from taking the medicines, I knew they were my only chance at living, and so I took them faithfully.

Summer and fall 1997 were also the first time I fully realized the power of our story in helping others see the possibilities for life and for their own relationships with God. We had been consumed with our own struggle for so long that we were unprepared for how our story touched others' lives. But in one way after another, God provided opportunities for us to give our testimony in churches and other settings. I also began to speak more openly in sermons, until I reached a comfort level at which I included tidbits of our experiences here and there. We had spent years in survival mode, but as we shared our story, we discovered not only that it helped others — it helped us.

From those first times of sharing my story, God has brought me into contact with thousands of unique, needy people. I continue to watch in amazement as he uses my story, time and again, to say things that others cannot, or will not, say, even for their own lives and circumstances. I have watched as they have made connections with God that otherwise would not have found relevance. And I have watched as people from all theological, economic, and ideological backgrounds have found a common thread in *their* part of my story. None of us are without that broken edge, no matter how good, smart, or together we might think we are. I don't want to make more of our personal courage to tell the story than I should. We made a lot of mistakes before we caught on and were able to see the full ramifications of our own journey. At first we processed things only from one angle, not really tackling the ways we continued to disappoint God and each other, although we clearly knew that things were not okay. But God patiently met us in those places and used us anyway. However, nothing would compare with how it would feel to one day be totally free and only have the truth.

A HAPPY, HIGHLY PRODUCTIVE DRUNK

Several friends of mine have, at one time or another, been involved in a twelve-step program for addictions. On occasion I have taken parishioners, family members, and friends to the meetings myself, as a way of making sure that they attend regularly. Twelve-step programs can effect wonderful work in a person's life, to the extent the person attending them is willing to be healed.

One night I took a friend who had been going through a particularly bad bout with alcohol to one of the local meetings. He was a dangerous type of addict — happy and highly productive even while drinking. Once I convinced him to attend a meeting, his life quickly changed. After the first meeting, he was not very happy with me.

"I can't do this," he argued. "I can't talk about my life in front of those strangers."

"They won't be strangers long," I assured him. "And you need to tell this story. It is the only way you will get better."

Over the next weeks, he attended faithfully, and I met him afterward to talk. My friend was aware of the struggles in my life — the need to prove myself, my marital problems, the fears and struggles of putting on a happy face while I felt like I was dying on the inside. That particularly was more of a concern to my friend than any of the details he knew. As a recovering person, he understood the power of the spiritual attack I was under at the time. After one meeting we talked about his group, though he used no names. When he had finished talking about his own personal discoveries, he turned to me and my issues.

"You know," he told me, "you are a lot like those folks in that room. You know that, right?"

I was shocked by the analysis. I had been many things in my life, but I didn't have an addictive personality. "What do you mean?" I asked, a little defensive.

"Well, you've decided that you can do everything on your own, even if you pay lip service to your faith in God. Don't get me wrong, Shane; you're one of the nicest, best people I know. Hell, you've saved my life. But you're living like a happy, highly productive drunk: keeping it busy but not really feeling anything either."

I winced as the truth hit home.

He continued: "You know, I've learned two important things from these meetings. First, you can't move forward until you're ready to lay down the last drop of everything. Second, it will most probably get much worse before it gets better. I love you for what you have done for me, but I can see the weary look in your eyes. It's a sadness that I don't believe the Higher Power expects you to carry the rest of your life. Like drinking, if you don't set it down, eventually it'll be the end of you."

My friend's words hit me at the core of my life. His diagnosis was true. I had bottled my life into manageable parts. Pokey and I were living day to day, trying our best to savor the joyful moments, but we had no perspective, no way to see past our own junk to fully appreciate the possibilities. This was not the best that God wanted for us. We almost had everything going right, but *almost* wasn't enough.

A friend of mine uses this illustration: It would be ridiculous for us to travel 99 percent of the way home, only to stop at the mailbox and celebrate like a moron. The point is to make it *all the way* home. At the end of the day, it comes down to grace, for it is grace alone that can bridge the critical distance between our *almost* and *all the way*.

God was teaching me this the hard way in my health, my ministry, and my marriage. The 99 percent was not what would mark my success as a husband, father, or pastor; it was the last little part that would. I was careening to a halt against the simple fact that I was not enough. Grace, forgiveness, love, and faith—and not my own effort—would need to have the final say.

Pokey and I were just getting by as life chipped piece after tiny piece away from our perfect facade. This was a pattern, a cycle, and it wasn't something we could fix by working harder or better or smarter. Until the cycle was broken—and until we were willing to bear that cost—nothing would change. All we could do was hold on as the waves grew bigger, and trust that God still had more of our story to write.

Chapter 8

GLIMPSES OF A STRAIGHT LINE SO PRECIOUS

I buried my grandfather today. The service was beautiful. I stood by the grave site for what seemed an hour after everyone had left. I remembered how many times my grandfather and I had stood in grassy places and talked about things. I don't like death. But death is a part of living and marks why living should matter so much while we have it. The broken places remind us of why we crave being whole ... why it is so dear to us. It is our "crooked line" as C. S. Lewis would say, that makes glimpses of the "straight line" so precious.

—Journal entry, October 1997

After my parents' divorce when I was six years old, I lived the every-other-weekend syndrome. I visited my father every other weekend and at least two weeks in the summer. Any child of divorce recognizes the knot such a schedule ties in your gut. Navigating the pickups and drop-offs and hellos and good-byes — both physical and emotional — is something no child should bear. Throughout all of this, my grandfather was a shining light of consistent love.

Most Friday nights I could be found planted in front of Grandpa's television. Unlike my mom, he let me watch the "bad" shows — *Dukes of Hazzard*, *The Incredible Hulk*, and, my grandfather's favorite, *Dallas*.

When it was time to leave Grandpa's and return home, I would get physically ill. Without fail, my grandfather would always find me, usually lying on his bed.

"Okay, let's get up now. You know your mom will be so excited to see you," he'd say.

"But what about you? Won't you be sad?" I'd ask.

"Oh, yes, I'll be sad for a little while, but before I know it, it will be time for you to come back, and we'll have so much to talk about then."

From the beginning of my health issues, when the doctors told my family about my hemophilia, my grandfather understood best the difficult road I would walk. He wanted me to be cautious but not sheltered and never afraid to face my struggles.

He was affectionate and gentle, but he also had great expectations and could be quite the disciplinarian. No one shaped my view of the world more than my grandfather, and no one provided more of an example for how I wanted to live. I shared qualities of both my mother and father, but the only person I wanted to *be* was Grandpa.

My grandfather was a point of reference that reminded me of who I was and who I represented. As I grew up, he was always present for me, healthy and available. I was the one who moved around and got sick. So it came as a surprise when, in my twenties, he began dealing with several major health incidents, including heart surgery and an abdominal aneurysm. His health deteriorated rapidly, and there were several times we thought we would lose him.

Grandfather recovered, however — we even decided to play in a golf tournament together the last weekend in October 1997. It would be our first round of golf in almost two years.

My grandfather drove to town and bought new golf balls and a bag of new golf tees. He was excited about the tournament, but mostly, as he told the store clerk, he was excited about playing golf with his grandson. The day promised to be special. My grandfather also wanted to play well and "not embarrass" himself, so he decided to practice. It was an unusually hot day in October, even for Mississippi, as he began to hit ball after ball.

A quarter of an hour into his practice, he felt the first jolt of pains in his chest; his heart fluttered and he began to sweat. Chalking it up to the weather, he continued to practice. When the pain became more intense, he dropped his clubs and began to walk toward the clubhouse. Just as he reached it, he collapsed.

My father found him moments later and began CPR.

Grandpa's color was drained, and he had begun to bite his tongue, a natural seizure resulting from the body's reaction to what amounted to a systems shutdown. Someone called 911. When the ambulance arrived, my grandfather had been unconscious for nearly half an hour, and the damage to his brain and body was irreparable. The paramedics stabilized his heart's rhythm, but the muscle damage was significant.

My grandfather spent the next three days in a coma. The doctors informed us that little could be done, and he would likely pass away quite soon. One family member after another came to his bedside to say good-bye. When it was my turn, everyone else stepped out of the room until it was just me, my father, and my grandfather. I stood beside his bed looking at his still body. I took him by the hand and began to speak into his ear. I thanked him for the way he had loved and cared for me and for the example he had been to me.

Then I made him a promise. I told him that I would never forget what we had discussed on that hillside when I was sixteen years old. "I will never take one day for granted. To the end," I promised him, "no matter how difficult it becomes, I will never give up."

Standing to leave, I whispered his favorite line from Catherine Marshall's *A Man Called Peter*, a wonderful story about her husband, the former chaplain of the U.S. Senate. After suffering another major heart attack, and just as the ambulance was about to take him to the hospital, Marshall told his wife, "I will see you in the morning." Those were the last words Peter Marshall spoke.

Those words symbolized heaven to my grandfather. Heaven was always morning, and the light never ended. He had talked about heaven a lot over the previous months, about the joy of seeing his own mother and father again. He talked about visiting with old friends who had been lost in the war. To my grandfather, heaven was a new beginning; he'd seen a lot of dusk and darkness in his life, and he figured he was due for a sunrise or two.

"I will see you in the morning," I said, squeezing his hand and then kissing him on the forehead. "Save me a spot on that hillside—we'll have a lot to talk about by then."

My grandfather died later that evening.

ONE MORE GOOD-BYE

Just as I was working through my grandfather's death, another heartbreak happened, this time to another person I considered a rock in my life and to whom I credited much of my resilience in dealing with one crisis after another. As often happens in life, heartache piled on heartache until we wondered what to do next.

Since Pokey and I had returned to Mississippi, Nancy and I had reconnected. Nancy was more than my doctor; she became my cheerleader, friend, and encourager. Whenever Pokey and I faced a problem or difficulty, we called Nancy. She was more than aware of our marital problems, and in many ways, she became more of a physician to our souls than our bodies.

Over dinner one night, Nancy became more reflective than usual. She said, "You know I'm very proud of you. These troubles you and Pokey are facing can be overcome if you guys don't forget to focus on each other instead of everyone else. God has great things for you." At the time, I remember thinking that her words, and certainly her tone, sounded encouraging but also almost mournful.

"Nancy, is everything okay?"

"You bet!" she replied.

Everything was not fine. Nancy had been diagnosed with a mass in her chest that was attached to the chest wall. She died less than a month later.

I assisted with Nancy's funeral service. After the service, one person after another told me how much I had meant to Nancy, and that she had spoken of me often to friends and colleagues. I felt honored to have played such an important role in her life, especially knowing how many people had felt the same way about her. The words were comforting. Yet Nancy's loss seemed to lack any sense of meaning or purpose, and for the next several weeks, I found myself in very pointed conversations with God—when I was able to talk with him at all.

Several weeks after Nancy's death, I found a file that contained cards, letters, and notes I had saved from the days surrounding my ordination. In the file was a note from Nancy:

For Shane. Though the days seem long and difficult, here is my prayer for you: That you might not forget the possibilities and potential for each new day and that in wading through the sunsets and transitions of our lives, you might not forget that each day also holds a sunrise.

I was looking for the sunrise—somewhere, anywhere. It had been a long year—Pokey's needle stick, the death of my grandfather, and now Nancy's death. I needed a new view of the path. But God was peeling back the edges of our wounds one layer at a time, and I was about to confront something even more tragic than the losses we had previously encountered.

EMPTY PLACES

Just as my friend from the AA group predicted, things got worse before they got better. The next couple of years were very difficult. My grandfather's and Nancy's deaths broke my heart more painfully than anything I'd previously experienced. I consumed myself with work—and anytime I admitted to myself that I was staying busy to hide my pain, I worked even harder.

Pokey and I consider this period the toughest years of our marriage. Old scars throbbed and new wounds were agonizing. Looking back, that nearly unbearable pain was the starting point of God's healing. Each new ache pushed us toward a crossroads. Like us, God was tired of us living in the middle of good and bad, always caught between broken and whole.

Pokey and I found joy in parenting Sarai Grace. A couple of years later, we had another daughter, Juli Anna. The death of a friend's daughter in a sudden car accident had shaken us, and both Pokey and I decided to try for another child. We were in no shape to be having children, but if there was one thing we did well in our marriage, it was parenting, so we felt that, regardless of our marital status, another baby might actually bring us closer together. And she did. But even a new baby could not heal some of the wounds we had opened in each other.

My emotional abandonment of Pokey had triggered a myriad of poor decisions and responses in her. Like many who experience abuse at a young age, Pokey convinced herself that she was not pretty or good enough, especially when I made her feel that way through my attention being focused in other places, so she spent time looking for affirmation through unhealthy relationships. If the love of her life would not provide what she needed, she found the second best thing, and this person was more than willing to oblige. Pokey was convinced that she had fallen in love with this person and that he had done the same. However, as she would say later, she was still very much in love with me. Thus, Pokey spent years caught in the middle between the relationship she believed God wanted for her and the one that had appeared to take away the pain, loneliness, and grief. As Pokey would later tell in her own testimony, it was not anything that she wanted, but she felt it was the only thing she had.

My suspicions of the relationship grew over the years, but as I would confront her about the friendship, she would adamantly deny it. Of course, I realized that if my suspicions were true, Pokey was not the only one to blame. I knew that I missed the mark in many ways in my marriage and had allowed my affections for her to be clouded by other things, responsibilities, and people. I had spent so much time trying to do good Christian things that I missed the focus on the one most important covenant Christ gives us to model our relationship with God.

Thankfully, I realized what I had done and started going to a counselor to learn how to change the situation. Pokey would not go with me at this time, largely because, as she would describe later, she felt too guilty and was afraid that she would just confess. She was also heavily invested in the relationship with the friend, and the complexities of ending that relationship were now more than she knew how to handle. Keeping the balancing act going seemed to be her best option.

One day during one of our sessions, the counselor asked if I had prayed for God to humble me and to break Pokey's heart so that we could find our way back to each other. I did not understand what she meant. Again, I only had suspicions of what had been going on, but the counselor explained that for

Pokey to make her way back to me, God would have to break her heart and cause such a stir in her that only telling the truth and being 100 percent transparent with me would provide the kind of openness and honesty that could save our marriage. Then the counselor described that God would then need to humble me so completely that neither my pride nor my own guilt and anger would get in the way of accepting Pokey's confession. "Together," she said, "God will restore your marriage, but it will require as much from you as it will from her."

It took awhile for me to first pray that prayer. I was scared as to what it might actually mean. But I missed my wife, and I believe she was miserable and missed us too. So I began praying for God to intercede, to humble me and to break Pokey's heart.

Slowly, the cracks began. God provided several opportunities for us to take extended trips together and, for the first time in many years in our marriage, to have time to talk and truly focus on each other. Then God provided new, wonderful friends who helped model his grace along with his greater intentions for our marriage. But more important, God began to work in our spiritual connections to him and one another. We joined a small group and began doing Bible studies together. Little by little, God broke the pride and walls that had divided us. At the time, it didn't appear like much, but God was doing a remarkable work in us that would change our marriage, and our lives, forever.

During this time Pokey found the courage to break off the friendship with the other person. It was an extremely tough, emotional time for her. She was giving up the one thing she thought she had in order to risk getting back that which she believed was God's will for her life—our marriage. But she also knew it was a risk. She could not predict how I would react or if

I would be able to forgive and move on. And Pokey did not know what I had been praying. I had kept those prayers secret, because every time we would broach the issue, I could see the turmoil erupt in her and then in me. I even made friends with the other man in question in an attempt to see if what I feared was all just my imagination. Either I was a fool or under a cloud of grace, but that friendship seemed genuine from both sides, and on several occasions we met to pray together and talk about life's other issues. He was going through a spiritual awakening in his own life and, unknowing as I was, I became the spiritual mentor who helped him find his way into a relationship with Christ just as he was ending his relationship with Pokey. Looking back, the circumstances seem so strange that there is no doubt God's hand was involved.

It was an entirely unremarkable day when the final piece of the dam holding back the real brokenness in our marriage broke away, allowing the truth to flow forward. Pokey and I had attended a Bible study the evening before and had watched a wonderful video lesson on communication in marriage. We talked about the differences in what women and men need in a marriage. The next morning, as Pokey and I talked about the video at breakfast together, I could tell that something was on her mind. She made arrangements for Sarai Grace and Juli Anna to go to their grandparents. And she asked me to call into the office and tell them I would be late. She needed to talk to me about something. Later that morning, after getting the girls to their grandparents', I arrived back home to Pokey sitting on the edge of the bed. I could tell she was very nervous, as the blood appeared to have drained from her face. She patted for me to sit down beside her, and as she began to talk, emotion overwhelmed her and she began to cry.

"I need to tell you something," she said, sobbing. Her eyes were on the floor. "I'm not who you think I am."

"I'm confused," I muttered. And I was, deeply. Things had gotten better, and we were communicating more, almost like the old "Shane and Pokey." When she began talking, I was afraid of what would come next.

Then the dam broke. Pokey unloaded everything: the molestation at age seven, the broken life, the promiscuity as a teenager, the feeling of abandonment, an eating disorder, and then, finally, the inappropriate friendship. It had been going on for several years, and she had broken our marriage covenant. However, she had been praying that God would put us back together. She assured me that the relationship was now over and that she wanted to make our relationship work for real. Pokey gave as many details as she could, and the depth and length of the relationship were even more shocking than I had suspected. It all came out, like a person vomiting. The more she told me, the faster she talked. Her heart and voice began to race, and I could tell that she was unloading, for the first time, the heavy burdens that she had been carrying for these years by herself.

Finally, her body heaving with sobs, Pokey ran to the bathroom. She knelt by the toilet, throwing up for real again and again. I knelt beside her, trying to wipe her face with a cool cloth, but she kept pushing me away.

Finally, I put my arms around her and wouldn't let go.

She looked me in the eyes. "You can't love someone like me. It's too much."

Her sobs became more intense. I tried to hold her even more tightly, but she pulled away from me and stood up.

"I need to go, I need to go...."

She walked toward the bedroom door, and I followed her. I kept asking her to stop, and she kept walking, almost running toward the front door. I grabbed her from behind and held on to her. She stopped and said, "I can't do this anymore!"

Then she looked up at me with a serious look in her face and said, "Just take care of the girls...." I didn't know what she meant, but I couldn't take the time to find out. I grabbed her and pulled her into an embrace.

"I am not letting you go!"

As I continued to hold on, sobs shook her body. "It's too much," she repeated, "too much."

I held on for dear life.

Many minutes passed before Pokey put her face into my chest and stopped crying. We sat down on the floor by the door, and I held her for what seemed forever. Maybe for the first time in my life, I didn't say anything, despite my questions and the feeling of betrayal that was burning inside my chest like a constellation of pain. At that moment, Pokey was the most vulnerable and fragile person I had ever seen, and I was her husband. Taking care of her was the most important thing to me.

There was no way I was letting go.

It had been a decade since grandfather taught me that none of us choose to get up one day and "fight the monster." Instead, the monster finds us, and it's spoiling for a fight. What we *do* choose is whether to give up. People who have since learned of our marital struggles ask how we survived what experts say is an almost hopeless scenario. Our answer is simple: We define our chance for survival by God's rules.

It wasn't, and isn't, easy. One person after another suggested that we give in or give up. There was "too much water under the bridge" and "too much that seemed unforgivable."

In fact, as I liked to say, it wasn't about too much water under the bridge — our whole bridge was under the water! On top of all of the relationship issues, we still had my health issues, not to mention the baggage that continued to unpack itself in front of us. Each new issue revealed others until we felt overwhelmed; at some points, it did feel like too much, even with God at our side. Each time we thought we had done all we could, what remained was to stand.

And stand, we did. For what seemed like months, we worked on every angle of our relationship. We did everything that was humanly possible to save our marriage. But as each wound would heal, another one would pop open. I realized that as much as we wanted it to work, we were busy trying to put it all back together by ourselves. We had prayed for God to humble us and break our hearts. And he did. But we had then tried to work through the next stages without God. What we really needed was a new direction and a new beginning apart from the broken places we had been. As much as we wanted it to work for us, for our girls, and for God, we were out of ideas and, shockingly for a preacher, out of words. We needed a miracle.

EARL

By early 1999, the pain and difficulty of the previous year had worn me down, and I was contemplating asking for a sabbatical. Worse yet, most people had no idea how I was feeling. I kept putting on the happy face while dying on the inside. I wasn't able to think or get my mind around the things that were most important.

I learned that a ministers' group was holding a retreat in southwest Mississippi. The brochure billed the retreat as a renewal time for ministers. People would gather on a Monday evening and stay until Wednesday. There would be sessions for Bible study, fellowship, and some private time for reflection. It sounded like something I needed, at least to my friends and family.

I was more hesitant. My idea of getting away involves a five-star resort and a golf course. I agreed, however, and began to look forward to the time away—until I arrived, that is, and learned that it was a silent retreat. Silent retreats and I go together like peanut butter and pickles. I considered turning around and heading home, but I was too embarrassed.

I concluded that God had brought me to the retreat for a reason and that I would make the best of it. My optimism lasted about an hour. I was struggling with too many voices in my soul that both kept me from saying the things that needed to be said and also pushed me, at times, to say too much, especially to God. I wasn't confronting the things that would make me better, but kept harping on the things that only dragged me further into my pain. It was a long day and evening. I survived the first night by playing solitaire on my computer, hidden under the covers, of course.

Mornings at the retreat were an opportunity to share our prayer concerns aloud. I so dominated the group that my retreat brothers and sisters were growing antsy. The rest of the day was miserable. I was antagonistic and frustrated with the Bible studies. By the time dinner came around, I had taken my tray outside under a tree, refusing even to pray and bless the food. I just sat there angry at God, angry at myself, angry at the world.

What was I doing here? I thought. I went back to my room, packed my clothes, and sneaked out of the window because I was too ashamed to face anyone who might ask where I was going. I just got into my car and drove away.

A couple of miles from the retreat center was an old gas station and truck stop. I stopped to gas up, but the printer in the gas pump didn't print my receipt. For some reason, I felt like I needed to have it, so I moved my car closer to the store and walked inside.

The clerk was an older gentleman who was kind but moved slowly. He was more concerned with the chicken cooking in the fryer across the room than with my receipt, but finally he shuffled to the register. He apologized for the inconvenience of having to come inside and then asked if there would be anything else.

The chicken cooking in the corner smelled great. "Is the chicken ready?"

"Just a few more minutes," he said. "If you have time, you can sit in the booth and I'll bring you some out."

It was about 8:00 p.m., and we were alone. "Is it always this quiet?"

"Not usually," he replied. "Maybe it's the storm that's brewing. You know bad weather causes people to retreat and hunker down—kind of makes people act like fools." He smiled.

I understood what he meant, and for the first time, I smiled too. I knew what acting like a fool felt like. After all, I had just sneaked out the window at a silent retreat that was supposed to provide me some rest and peace.

I sat down at the booth and waited. The man brought out a huge basket of fried chicken and a Diet Coke.

Feeling the need to carry on a conversation after twenty-four hours of near silence, I said, "If you have a minute, you could sit and talk." He scooted into the seat across from me in the booth.

We sat there a minute until I finally asked, "So, what's your name?"

"Earl," he replied.

"That was my grandfather's name," I said.

"Were you close?" the man asked.

"Very close," I said, continuing to eat my chicken. "He passed away about a year ago." I stopped talking because I could feel the lump in my throat.

"I'm sorry to hear that," he answered. "You up here for business or for pleasure?"

"Well, I guess it was both," I replied. I put down my chicken, almost embarrassed by the question and certainly by the answer. I didn't know this man, but he seemed oddly familiar, and since I had not talked to anyone in over twenty-four hours, I let down my usual barriers and started to talk.

"I was here for a retreat, but that didn't work out so well," I said. "My family thought it would be good for me. I just lost a dear friend, and it's been a long year. I think my congregation was getting worried about me too."

"Congregation?" the man asked. "You a preacher?"

"Yes," I answered, feeling particularly unqualified for the job.

"So, you were staying at the retreat center just up the road?" he inquired.

"Yes," I said. "It's a nice place, but the retreat was a silent retreat, and ... well, I just got tired of being quiet, I guess." I had turned by now and was looking out the windows to the gas pumps.

"Well, sport, that seems like a good reason to leave."

"What did you say?" I asked quickly. No one had called me "sport" since my grandfather died.

"I said that seems like a good reason to leave," he said. "No one should be at a silent retreat if they don't want to be quiet." I could tell he was puzzled by my reaction.

"Yes, I guess it is," I said shyly, trying to gauge whether this was all real or I was imagining the conversation now.

"Does being quiet scare you or something?" the man asked.

"Not usually," I said. "But lately, I don't really know what pushes my buttons anymore. All I know is that being quiet didn't do it for me."

"So you snuck out?" he asked.

"Yes," I said warily. "How'd you know that?"

"Well, no offense," he offered. "But you look like someone who's either running from something chasing you or sneaking away from something you don't want to confront."

Actually, I was doing both at the same time. I was being chased by the pain, grief, and disappointment of the past months but also afraid to face the complete surrender that God needed if I was to be healed. I sat back, wondering if Earl was really a store clerk or some divine spiritual agent sent to prevent my escape from the silent retreat. Either way, I was listening now.

"What if it's both?" I asked.

"Well, then," Earl answered, "I would suspect that you are really tired."

I *was* tired. In fact, I was exhausted and alone. I felt as if I had to have all of the answers, as if I had to be some special conduit from "on high," even when I didn't feel plugged into anything myself. I was tired of trying to make sense of things and of trying to appear strong. I didn't feel strong; I didn't feel spiritual; and I didn't feel inspired.

I was tired of being tired.

Earl and I talked for nearly two hours. I shared my story with him, the ups and downs and the sense of emptiness I felt trying to do it all myself.

"Well, that seems to be your problem, right there," he said. "You spend most of your time trying to being so many things to so many people that you miss being the one thing you were meant to be in the first place."

"And what would that be?" I asked.

"His, Shane, simply his," he answered, this time quiet and pastoral. For a moment, I felt as though I were talking to my grandfather again.

"I don't know where to start," I said to Earl.

"How does the beginning sound?" Earl replied.

The beginning. It sounded so simple. Could I just go back and surrender? Could I lay it all at God's feet? Could I trust that he could work in my pain? I asked Earl these questions.

"The real question is, will you?" Earl said.

I leaned my chin on my fist, now balanced on the table. "Well, the problem —" I began, the lump in my throat getting deeper. "I can't pray right now," I finally mumbled, tears now filling my eyes. "I can't pray...."

"Then let me pray for you," Earl said. Taking my hand in his, Earl prayed. It was a simple request. "Help there to be less of Shane and more of you in his life, Lord. He doesn't need to do what he has never been built to do. Be all that and more for him. You don't break your promises. Thank you."

I left the truck stop and drove back through the darkness to the silent retreat. *The steadfast love of God never ceases,* I thought, *and his mercies are new every morning.* I looked forward to the rising sun — to a new day when I could truly, by God's grace, begin again.

Just then I was glad for the darkness, however; I still needed to sneak back into my room. I had not expected it, but nonetheless, I had found my miracle at the truck stop with my new friend Earl.

At the same time, Pokey was finding her own miracle at a Beth Moore conference. God asked Pokey a similar question as Earl asked me, "If I could look into your heart, would I be pleased?" Pokey knew that God would be pleased with parts and not pleased with others. She had done everything but turn over the collateral damage of the last years to him. She had not turned over the shame and guilt and had tried fixing and bearing those burdens on her own. She had survived the onslaught of the truth and confession but was dying under the weight of putting the pieces back together again.

Our issue now was not the secrets or deception, but whether we would give God control of our lives. While I was answering the question with my new friend at the truck stop, Pokey found friends of our own gathered around in prayer for her at the conference, and though many of them had no idea about the details, they prayed a new breath into this broken woman.

When I arrived home, I found a different person than before, and I knew that Pokey had spent some serious quality time with God. Certainly all of our questions weren't answered or all the hurts fixed. But we had turned over the direction of our struggle to the One who could make the serious difference. And in return, we not only found our marriage again, but we found peace when confronting the most difficult issues between a husband and wife. Most important, we learned how to love each other again, not with our own wisdom or strength, but by seeing each other as Christ sees us — warts and all.

Pokey and I continued to work hard on our issues and on past hurts. We reworked every direction of our lives and retooled our priorities to put each other first. It was not always an easy road, and at times the details became very complicated. But we held on to each other by holding on to God and saw the end of the tunnel and were amazed by the light and new beginning.

Out of respect for our daughters, we do not talk much about this period of our lives. Some will ask why we even included something so personal in this book. The answer is simple: We have watched many people walk down a similar path and give up. We have seen couples get to a point in their marriages where they believed God could not come through on his promise to heal their brokenness and put them back together again. After much prayer, Pokey and I believed we owed it as a testimony and witness to God for our own marriage to tell the story and say unequivocally and unashamedly that not only does God keep his promises, but life is so much sweeter when we discover that he does.

Several years later, when sharing our testimony at a marriage retreat, Pokey told the story from John 8 of the woman caught in adultery. When she is about to be stoned, Jesus steps in and asks, "Where are your accusers, daughter?" Pokey heard these words in her own heart and could only answer, like the woman in the biblical account, in one way: "Nowhere."

Just as Jesus answered the woman, he answered Pokey.

"Then neither do I accuse you. Get up and start again. The rocks prepared for condemnation lie in the dirt; step over them and continue down the road. The rocks can't hurt you now."

Pokey is the most precious person I have ever known. She is the best mother a man could ask to watch over their children and the dearest friend I could ever imagine. And though it may seem odd to others, realizing the sweetness of where we have landed, I wouldn't change a thing if it meant missing out on what we have now. Of course, I wish we would have learned these lessons before the pain and wasted days, but when I look into the eyes of my wife and best friend now, I see a beautiful daughter of God who doesn't carry the shame and burden of life any longer, and whose heart and life are restored and redeemed. The love of my life has long since stood up from the dirt and brushed herself off, and she is beautiful to behold.

SWEET VOWS ONCE MORE

A couple of years later, Pokey and I, now the parents of three beautiful girls, decided to renew our marriage vows. We had experienced vast healing and renewal, and we wanted to say to God, each other, our daughters, and others that we cherished our newfound beginning.

We decided to hold the ceremony in the new worship chapel at Duke Divinity School. It was a beautiful setting. Our families, who had experienced so much angst during the planning of our first wedding, were relaxed and enjoyed the time together. And the girls, who knew very little as to why we would renew our vows, just saw the time as their mother and father saying how much they loved each other and their girls.

Pokey bought a new dress, and I surprised her with a new engagement ring and a new wedding band. The old ring, which represented old days and other promises, was made into a pendant that Pokey wears around her neck. And we even were able to arrange for a dear friend at Duke to officiate at the vows.

It was a beautiful time, and once again, as Pokey arrived in her new dress, she took my breath away. Of course, we were different, too, this time. We had been through the fire and had survived, and life was more than a collection of days for us; it was a chance to make the best of every moment. We wouldn't take it for granted this time around.

Chapter 9

A MATTER OF THE HEART

I placed the final period in place and sat back to look at the screen. It was the last period in the last sentence of the last page of the first book I had ever written.* I thought I would feel different, maybe caught up in the moment. But nothing. It was another day. Another project finished. The only thing to do was what I had done all of my life—move on to the next project, place, or issue. Doesn't sound like much, but it is what I know and what keeps me going.

—Journal entry, March 2005

**The Seven Next Words of Christ: Finding Hope in the Resurrection Sayings* (Nashville: Abingdon Press, 2006).

A neighbor of mine has a '68 El Camino. He bought the car because it belonged to his father who died of cancer. The car reminds my neighbor of his dad, and the vehicle possesses a deep sentimental value—a value sometimes hidden to others behind the layers of rust and peeling paint. If you ask my neighbor why he keeps the car, he answers, "Oh, it ain't much, but it's mine."

For many years I felt the same about life—"It ain't much, but it's mine." Yet my life had much more value than I knew or appreciated. Once God cleared the storm clouds from our view, Pokey and I rediscovered a life filled with possibilities and opportunities, not just in our marriage and family, but also in the ways that God was providing for us to share our story with others, serve in ministry together, and make a difference in our world. The road wasn't any easier now; the difference was that we were walking it together. And as we continued to heal, God provided new friends and physicians to help along the way.

My complicated medical conditions—hemophilia as well as HIV/AIDS—continued to be a challenge. For me to wake up with a spontaneous bleed in an elbow or ankle was not uncommon. I undertook a special diet and training schedule to help with flexibility and conditioning, but there were no guarantees that the next morning I wouldn't wake up with a locked elbow or knee joint.

And along with HIV/AIDS and hemophilia, I continued to wrestle with hepatitis C, a slow-moving disease that I will eventually have to confront more fully. For the moment, it is held in check with a medicine that causes me to feel like I have the flu for days at a time. Interestingly, given the many times I have discussed my HIV status, I have had just as much response from people about hep C. Hundreds of people have contacted me to disclose their status *for the first time*, perhaps seeing me as the only safe person to tell. I recently received an email from a pastor who also deals with HIV and hep C but had not told his family or his congregation. He wrote that he had decided to share the news, first with his loved ones and then with his parishioners. He wrote later to inform me that he had told both his family and his congregation. "It was tough but obviously the right thing to do," he said, adding that it felt good "not to live with the burden alone" any longer.

Over the years, I have witnessed the inner workings of the Community of the Chronically Ill, as I call it. I am not saying that others necessarily have the same struggles as I or vice versa, but people who live with disease or illness gain a different perspective about life. Living with disease unveils the strange ebb and flow of human nature, expectation, and possibility in the one dealing with the disease or illness and in the ones with whom he or she comes into contact. Some of the worst of humanity I have ever witnessed is connected to HIV/AIDS. Yet some of the finest acts of altruism and simple charity have been due to the fight in this arena, where no other bridge could be found. Chronic illness provides little middle ground. People respond either from their fear or from their courage. I have witnessed various friends who could not overcome the stereotypes surrounding my own disease or the issues that surrounded it, and we have since lost touch. But I have also seen other friends, who some would think least likely to reach out, become the best advocates a person with this disease could have. The difference is found in relationships. When people know someone who connects them specifically to the disease, their approach is dramatically different from that of people who have no connection. Either way, for those of us in my family and especially my close friends, the disease always served as a compass for our priorities and expectations in the world. Often it is not so much that we keep the disease in check, but that the disease keeps *us* in check—reminding us that what divides us is, ultimately, of little consequence.

NEW VOICES

As Pokey and I grew healthier, we realized how much we wanted to have more children. Emma Leigh was born in March 2004. Although we went for years planning our life without children, it is impossible now to imagine life without them! Our girls complement our life as a couple and as individuals. The responsibility of caring for another life and for setting an example, knowing that how you live your life models how a child will also see and respond to the world, is enormous. As significant as our accomplishments in our respective careers, Pokey and I agree that we have no more important job than being the best parents we can be. But our roles as parents also carry over to our walk for Christ in general.

Pokey and I realized that part of us getting our marriage right and living faithfully was about how our own children as well as others would see us live our lives. We wanted them to find in us examples of people who took the struggles, difficulties, and opportunities of life and made a difference, both by responding by doing our best with our God-given gifts, but also with a sense of humility, knowing that only God could complete the "good work" in us.

The older I get, the more I think about the example my mother set raising a sick child, and about her own faithfulness to do her best in spite of what seemed unbelievable odds. I remember her life centered around joy, worship, devotion, and especially prayer. My mother prays beautiful, sweet-spirited, prayers. She doesn't just talk to God—she walks into God's presence and sits down for a visit. I can always tell when my mother has been praying. The look on her face speaks to having been in the presence of power, majesty, and love. She *is* how she *prays*. I learned to pray by watching my mother. She paid attention to the example she was setting, and I am the better for it.

For Pokey and me, healing from the wounds, struggles, and obstacles of our lives was not enough. We needed to "be" something else, too, for ourselves, for our children, and for those who would watch our example, even when we didn't know it. God expected that from us.

With all of the diseases and difficult paths, God was placing a plan for our lives in front of us and then unfolding it piece by piece. We had been through many "toils and snares," as the old hymn says, but we had done more than survive; we had prevailed. But now our responsibility was to live out what God had done for us, what God had taught us to trust and be. To whom much is given—and Pokey and I have received countless blessings—much is expected. And we were only just about to start giving back.

TRANSITIONS

God taught us volumes about himself during our time at Asbury. The church truly exhibited the Spirit as the living, breathing

Body of Christ, from worship to fellowship to missions. Many of my friends in ministry would remark, "You know, you could stay at Asbury forever."

Looking back, they were right. I had been offered new opportunities at various times through the course of my ministry at Asbury, but it never seemed to be the right time to leave. However, in the spring of 2004, I could tell that God was doing something unique. The United Methodist Foundation approached me about leading a new project that would develop stewardship and healthy church programs and assessments for over eleven hundred United Methodist churches. We had certainly come a long way from discussing whether I could be appointed to a local church!

At first I turned down the offer, citing my continued work at Asbury and my ever-growing ministry beyond its walls. I was traveling to congregations across the country and discovering that my contribution to their church life involved more than the story of my health journey. They needed new concepts for how to relate in an ever-changing world.

Many of the churches experienced the type of dynamics that experts call "acoustic shadows." This is a phenomenon in war when locals not far from a battle cannot hear the war at their doorsteps, while others miles and miles away can hear every shot and every mortar round. What the term means for churches leaders is that oftentimes the closer we are to a congregation, the harder it is to hear and see the needs and struggles. Many times a person from the outside provides a much more objective view and assessment. One of my gifts in this new role was to "hear the sounds of a church's battle" and to relay those dynamics to the church. Many churches are unprepared to make changes regarding worship styles, serving others — especially the marginalized and under-resourced — and the spiritual values of the next generation. And with many congregations caught in a strictly institutional mind-set, the ability to shake the chains of the institution and approach faith from a fresh, flexible point of view is difficult. Of course, in reality "institutional mind-set" affects every aspect of a church's life, including its resources and growth. But ultimately the conversation is about change and about being able to face difficult conversations head-on.

Maybe that is why I found myself so able to hold these conversations with churches. First, change did not scare me. I had faced it my whole life, from my health especially. I was able to confront difficult conversations with an objective nature of where to proceed — not that many of the conversations in the churches were about having your marriage come apart at the seams or finding out that you have a terminal illness. Mainly my job, mostly fashioned from my journey, was about getting people to stop and take an assessment of what was important and what was not. To that end, a person with a chronic illness makes a great church health consultant.

And I was broadening my ministry into other areas of communication, including writing. I had written a couple of articles for two national denominational magazines about "ministry horizons" and effective stewardship and had received very positive reviews. The thought of working and consulting full-time had crossed my mind, but I didn't have a clear view of what that might look like.

When the United Methodist Foundation approached me a second time about the position, the Lord sent one sign after another that I needed to accept their offer. I had moved beyond

U.S. Postal Service fleeces by this point, but every marker I used for discerning God's will pointed to this new direction in my life. Although I couldn't see why God would lead me in this new direction, I wasn't about to question him after everything I had witnessed over the past few years. Whatever God had up his sleeve for tomorrow, I would try to simply be faithful enough to trust him today. With a willingness to be surprised, I accepted the United Methodist Foundation's offer to lead their ministries for Stewardship and Church Health.

Surprised I was. Over the next three years, God opened doors that, just a few years earlier, would have seemed locked forever. I spoke at the Saddleback Global AIDS Summit in California. I joined the staff of the *United Methodist Hour*, a thirty-five-year-old television and radio ministry primarily seen on stations throughout Mississippi, Tennessee, and Arkansas. When I became host of the program in 2006, we joined the FamilyNet broadcast schedule, and overnight the program went from airing in 3 million homes to more than 30 million homes in forty-eight states. The HIV positive pastor, who fifteen years earlier was afraid to speak about his condition, now had the privilege of sharing with millions of people each week.

One of the most special developments in my ministry was the creation of the Maji Project. The program provides rehydration kits for children suffering from dehydration and HIV. Originally the idea of our daughter Sarai Grace, who had seen a news report on the lack of drinking water for children in sub-Saharan Africa, the project has provided water to more than twenty thousand children in just two years. This little program born from a simple idea resonates the philosophy a dear friend once mentioned to me: "We may not be able to do everything, but we can do something—and when everyone is doing something, anything is possible." This saying was more than just the slogan of our water rehydration project; it had become a description for our life and ministry.

In the midst of all of these changes, we continued to travel, write, and speak. Pokey's career also blossomed, and God had indeed expanded our boundaries beyond our wildest imaginations. Pokey traveled across the United States teaching seminars and continuing education through the Bureau of Educational Research. And I continued to speak at church and business events, sharing my journey. The pace was quick and, at times, difficult. But we loved it as it gave us a chance to make a difference. Through letters, our website, and email, people were sharing their stories, so we knew that God was using each event, speech, and seminar to awaken people to a new way of viewing life.

My health remained stable. I had been on the same medicines for several years, and I functioned at a high standard with them. I felt fatigued at times and knew that I had to eat right and exercise to keep the side effects under control, but everything seemed in order. And so I lived happily ever after and, one day, I wrote a book about it all.

Well, not exactly.

A MATTER OF THE HEART

Just when we thought life had become manageable and we understood all of its twists and turns—well, life happened again. One day while working out, I experienced a strange sensation in my chest. Tests revealed a 98 percent blockage in one of the main arteries to my heart. The doctors' nickname for this type of blockage is "the widow maker," because most people don't catch it in time, and it usually results in a sudden cardiac arrest.

The only way to correct the blockage was a single bypass procedure that would take the mammary artery from my chest wall and move it into the place of the blocked artery. Of course, the surgery, already critical and complicated, was intensified by my hemophilia and other conditions. In fact, so few hemophiliacs had such a procedure that no doctor could say for sure what the odds of success might be. The only certainty shared by each doctor was that doing nothing would most likely mean sudden death.

Pokey and I were stunned. This wasn't on our radar, and it took some time to get our bearings. Not having the surgery was clearly not an option—I had too much to live for, so not doing anything was out of the question.

But the cure was no sugar pill; it was quite possible that the surgery or the recovery would kill me. Thus it was that on Good Friday 2007 I checked into the hospital for observation in preparation for surgery the following Monday.

It was a difficult weekend. I had prepared myself for so many things, but this caught me off guard. One of the ways I had fought my health struggles over the years was in not dwelling on the condition, always assuming things would turn out well. Given the gravity of this situation, however, I needed to say things to my daughters and Pokey, just in case. But the words wouldn't come. I couldn't bring myself to say what I needed to say, and I realized that I was under a spiritual attack.

Of course, Pokey and I had been there before, and we knew the only way to confront a spiritual battle like this was to face

Satan head-on. That Saturday night, we had a long conversation in which we audibly challenged the demons that surrounded our lives, and we specifically claimed the promises of God. It was a tough time, but one that also drew Pokey and me even closer. I told her that I might not survive the procedure, but we were certainly not going to spend the next days living in fear. Pokey prayed the sweetest, most honest prayer that thanked God for all we had been through. She asked for a safe procedure and for healing, but she also asked for strength, joy, and wisdom in *however* we saw God's hand working in our lives over the next days.

After the prayer, Pokey climbed into the hospital bed with me, and we just lay there holding each other. I had held her at so many other difficult times, but this time we held each other without any secrets or without regrets. We knew that these next moments might be our last together, and we wanted to hold each other for as long as we could. Pokey fell asleep. I could feel the gentle movement of her breathing. Finally, I fell asleep, too, and we stayed there until a nurse woke us the next morning.

The next day, Pokey and the girls attended Easter services at the church where I had been teaching part-time. The worship leader led them in a chorus that talked about the power of God. "My Savior, he can move the mountains. \ My God is mighty to save." As Pokey and the girls sang, tears filled their eyes, and Emma Leigh looked up and asked, "Will God be able to save our daddy?"

"Yes," Pokey said, not knowing if God would save me physically or by calling me home to that everlasting sunrise where Grandpa Earl was waiting for me.

Later that day, the girls arrived at the hospital room. We shared a wonderful afternoon of Easter bunny goodies. (How had he known to bring their baskets to my hospital room instead of to the house?) By the time they got ready to leave, I knew I wanted to say several things to them. Many emotions were going through my heart, but mainly I wanted them to know how much I loved them and how proud I was to be their father.

I took each one of them in my arms, hugged and kissed them, and then whispered words of love and hope in their small ears. Juli Anna and Emma Leigh did not know quite what to make of it all, but Sarai Grace, by this time ten, understood. In the sweetest manner, she reached back and hugged me again and said, "I am proud of you, too, Daddy. . . . I'm proud of you."

When they left the room, I broke down and wept, partially because of the situation, but also out of joy in knowing that God had blessed me with such wonderful children. I would prefer to watch them grow up, but if that moment were my last, it was as complete a feeling of confidence in who they were as any parent could have had.

The next morning an overwhelming number of friends and family arrived in my hospital room. Pokey did her best to keep things as normal as possible, putting most of her focus on me, but I knew the situation was very stressful for her. Eventually the doctors arrived to take me to the operating room. They wheeled me away, allowing Pokey to walk by my side. I passed the faces of loved ones and felt blessed to be loved by so many people. The last face along the line was that of my mother. She had long since passed the mantle of my primary care over to Pokey. However, as a parent now myself, I can imagine her feelings. We had never been much for public displays of affection, though I knew very well that she loved me, but as the gurney went past, she stopped it and kissed me on the forehead. I could tell that she was very upset, but as she wiped away tears, she whispered into my ear how proud she was of me and how much she loved me. I told her I loved her too, and we moved on through the doors.

We arrived in pre-op and were met by doctors and nurses getting their supplies together for the procedure. It was a hectic scene, yet every last one took the time to stop and tell me he or she was praying for me. Their personal care almost made me forget, for a moment, what we were facing.

Finally, the doctors gave me something to make me drowsy. I could still feel the touch of Pokey's hand as she continued to stroke my face. She leaned down every few moments to kiss me on the forehead. Finally, as nurses informed her that it was time, she leaned down and whispered "I love you" in my ear.

I looked up at her and said my last audible words before drifting off to sleep: "I love you."

Before I lost consciousness, however, I spoke silently to one other person. "If this is the time when I am supposed to see you, I am ready. You are my Lord, my Savior, and my Friend, and I trust you."

I drifted off to sleep.

Chapter 10

THE FIRST DAY
OF THE REST OF MY LIFE

This is the first time I have journaled since having surgery. I have a port in me, strapped to a pump that is an endless flow of Factor. My body hurts. But I am here. I survived. I have spent most of the day watching the Food Network. Don't ask me why. I don't cook very well and certainly will never at the level of those guys. Funny what gets your attention when you are flat on your back.

—Journal entry, April 12, 2007

It is wrong to take friends and life for granted, and I am the chief among sinners. We never travel our road alone, and it's never too late to put an arm around the shoulders of those who walk beside us. The deeper our relationships, the deeper our connection to God.

Many in our world live the lie of self-sufficiency — a lie that we have believed from the beginning. We choose, too often, to believe that we can be enough, despite all evidence to the contrary. My grandmother, a child of the Depression, passed along this wisdom directly and often. She would always say, "Boy, you're smart, but you will never be smart enough." She knew there would always be something bigger than me, something I couldn't accomplish on my own, no matter how successful I was.

Knowing that we can never save ourselves or our families can cause despair; paradoxically, it can also nourish hope, for it is in our weaknesses that God's strength is made perfect.

WAKING UP

I had been told prior to surgery that when I woke up I might have strange sensations related to pain and the discomfort of my ventilator. I was told that although I might want to panic, I was to try to stay calm. I laughed this advice off — what was I listening to, a flight attendant doing the safety spiel?

What I did fear was waking up alone.

As predicted, I woke to the awkward feeling of something in my throat and to waves of pain as well. But at the same time, I heard voices. The sweet voice of my wife called my name. I could feel her stroke my face, and I could smell her perfume. The next voice I heard was of my best friend, Ronnie. Hearing his voice gave me a great sense of calm. "Shane, you did great!" he said. His voice was followed by the voices of other friends and family.

I was listening to a chorus of angels; I was the farthest thing from alone.

God didn't create us for isolation. We are made to live life together. Community allows us to take in the full breath of fellowship and friendship, making us more alive as individuals than ever. We are created in God's image — our triune God who is Father, Son, and Spirit.

During the weeks following surgery, I experienced the most tangible expressions of God's presence I have ever felt. Of course, we had our ups and downs. I had several setbacks with my wound, and the pain — even for a guy who was used to having trouble healing — was excruciating.

Four weeks into my recovery, my insurance administrator called me and informed me that, because of the high cost of the Factor, I had met my lifetime maximum for health insurance coverage. I thought I was going to have a heart attack. The nurse administrator informed me that I would need to make other arrangements for payment of medical services.

"Other arrangements?" I asked.

"Yes," she said. "You will need to make personal arrangements to cover the cost of medical services from this point on."

"But ma'am," I replied, "I am just out of surgery. What do I do?"

"There are several options for assistance programs and Medicaid. I'll send them in the mail."

In the mail? I was over my insurance limit by hundreds of thousands of dollars with no means to pay it back. "God," I prayed, "am I going to survive open heart surgery but die from lack of funds?"

Thankfully, through the skilled workings of a wonderful man named David Stotts, the insurance maximum was raised by another one million dollars. As much as I would like to think it was for me, the plan had been in the works for some time. The lifetime maximum had been too low as people began to live longer. Within weeks of this news, the United Methodist Church in Mississippi (the organization funding my health insurance) raised the maximum benefit for my health insurance. It was a miracle with perfect timing. Without it, I would not have been able to afford the other costs associated with recovery.

I was able to negotiate, through the help of two dear friends who worked for the hospital, a significant reduction in my bill. But it sent a shockwave through me to consider the huge cost of staying alive. How blessed I was that I had the means and availability of coverage. I don't take such coverage or benefits for granted now, and I never will.

Heart surgery reminded me that my life was an opportunity that I never want to take for granted. My life isn't simply about my own journey — it provides a connecting path with many other roads. For example, during the 2007 World AIDS Day, I keynoted an event with Jeanne White, the mother of AIDS activist Ryan White. Over the course of those two days, we shared several stories of living with and through the disease. I was amazed at the struggle of those early days. She was amazed at how far I had come in the years since I had gone public.

As we parted after the conference, Jeanne turned to me and said, "Ryan would have been just a year or so younger than you now." The words stopped me in my tracks. This young boy, whom we all remember for his youth, strength, and courage, would have been in his late thirties now.

Jeanne is very humble and quiet, except when she is talking about Ryan. His life and struggle had made it possible, through the Ryan White legislation sponsored by Senator Ted Kennedy, for people with HIV and other chronic illnesses to afford medical care. I realized how much I owed to Ryan and to his life, and I shared that with Jeanne.

"He would have liked your life," Jeanne said. "He would have liked your life very much." Her words reminded me that I liked my life too. My life, in all its struggles and successes, was blessed beyond words. Many, hearing of my circumstances, wonder how I can say that I have lived a charmed life. I wonder how I could think otherwise.

GULF BREEZE

Remember Larry Goodpaster? The former chair of the Board of Ministry who had met clandestinely with Pokey and me in the hotel room nearly fifteen years earlier had been elected as a bishop in the United Methodist Church in 2000. In the fall of 2008, Larry was working to appoint a senior pastor at Gulf Breeze United Methodist Church, one of the largest UM churches in the country. The congregation had been served by the same pastor for nearly twenty-five years, and Herb was now serving as interim leader until a permanent replacement could be found.

Bishop Goodpaster called me on a Tuesday afternoon. We

had not spoken for almost seven years. "I have been praying about who will be the next leader of the church," he said, "and your name keeps coming to mind."

I was dumbfounded. Was God leading us in a new direction again? What about my current ministries? Gulf Breeze had more than five thousand members! With all these thoughts racing through my head, all I could manage to say was, "My name?"

"Yes," chuckled Larry, "your name."

How far it seemed from that hotel room in North Carolina to this conversation! When the interim senior pastor, Herb Sadler, called a few days later, I was honest about my contentment with my current life, and I was also forthright about my health and my story.

"We know all about that," Herb said. "I don't think anyone will see that as a problem."

I couldn't help but laugh.

Over the next weeks, Herb and I talked several times. He introduced key members of the congregation to my website, and several of them began subscribing to my podcasts and reading one or more of my books. I had written two more books since *The Seven Next Words* in 2006: *The Eight Blessings* in 2007 and *When God Disappears* in 2008.*

"You're the one!" Herb said during one of our phone calls. "*We've* decided — now it's just a matter of convincing *you* and the powers that be."

He wasn't talking about UMC powers. Moving Pokey from her house and from the community that had provided so much

---

The Eight Blessings: Recovering the Beatitudes (Nashville: Abingdon Press, 2007) and *When God Disappears: Finding Hope When Your Circumstances Seem Impossible* (Ventura, CA: Regal Books, 2008).

safety seemed almost impossible. Now that the girls were getting older, taking them from their network of friends became even more complicated. Pokey and I prayed about the decision and basically left it in God's hands: *If this is your will, then open the doors. But if not, Lord, please shut them tight and throw away the keys!*

Our first glimpse of God's intentions was Sarai Grace's prayer one evening when she thanked God for "giving us patience to trust in him instead of our own wants and desires." The next sign were the people of Gulf Breeze. From the first meeting, our conversations and interactions were blessed with hospitality and grace. By the end of our trip, the family took a vote, and it was unanimous. Of course, this was all very scary — leaving our home, our friends, our doctors, and the community we had grown to love. And of course, our friends found it hilarious that the one person they knew who did not like sun, sand, and water was going to pastor a church surrounded by sun, sand, and water.

God called, we answered, and once again we witnessed — and are witnesses to — the creative love of a God of new possibilities. At Gulf Breeze we discovered a congregation infused with compassion, love, and a vision for healing people. Our church motto is "Hope, hospitality and healing in the name of Jesus Christ." One church member, after reading my story and meeting me and my family, said with a grin, "If there's anyone whose life symbolizes our motto, it's you!"

Chapter 11

WHAT HAPPENS NEXT, DADDY?

I started combining the sermon files and catalogs from the past fifteen years to get ready for the move and was shocked to discover that I had 1,031 sermons in various files. However, when I categorized the topics, most (over 600) of the sermons can be traced to sermons preached from one of three gospel passages about the love and forgiveness of Jesus. No hard topics, no controversial issues—just the love of Jesus preached from a few Scriptures. Did I preach so many from one place because the people needed it or because I did? Either way, the gospel is simple and profound if we stay with the most important thing he said.

—Journal entry, June 2009

In our house, you can't watch PG movies until you have turned ten years old. It is a big date and one that is longed for and, when achieved, much celebrated. When our oldest daughter, Sarai Grace, turned ten, the first PG movie she wanted to see was *Star Wars*. It was and is one of my favorites.

When I was younger than Sarai Grace, my grandfather took me to the local theater in the small town where we lived to see the premiere of George Lucas's new, exciting space drama. I remember watching half of the movie with my head buried in my grandfather's shoulder, looking up only enough to ask, "What happens next?"

By the time Sarai Grace and I sat down to watch the movie, I had prepared her for the vast cast of characters, including Darth Vader and all of the others who would be far more unnerving than anything she had seen before. She assured me that she was now big enough to handle the movie and that she was ready. I said okay and put the DVD in the player.

Within the first ten minutes, or somewhere around the first time we met the Sith Lord, Sarai Grace, much like me years earlier, had buried her face in my shoulder. She looked up occasionally, when the silence overtook the pounding music, and asked, "What happens next, Daddy?" My response was always, "You will have to watch and see, sweetie."

It is not uncommon for children of any age, size, or disposition to ask that question. It is also not uncommon for God's children to do the same thing. I know that I have reached a certain place in my life where I would love a blueprint for what comes next around the corner. However, my Father responds much as I did for Sarai Grace: "Watch and see."

SERMONS, CHANCELS, AND OLD ROADS

A few weeks ago, I preached my first sermon as the new senior pastor of Gulf Breeze United Methodist Church. I preached about Shadrach, Meshach, and Abednego, the famed characters who marched to the fire for their faith in Daniel 3. It was a good day, filled with the busyness of three sermons, countless questions and decisions, and meeting as many people as possible.

After the service was finished and most of the worshipers had made their way to Sunday lunch, I walked back into the sanctuary and sat on the steps leading up to the chancel area. I looked back down the long center aisle of the sanctuary and reflected on the day. This was another chapter in my life, another twist in the path. God is always doing something new, and lately it seemed as though God had been doing new things more and more often.

This can be disorienting, yet it is the next day — the next bend in the road — that shows us what we cannot see from where we are now. If we are faithful enough to follow, we discover that God is in control, no matter how out of control we feel. Does that mean everything works in perfect accordance with our hopes and dreams? Absolutely not. I never dreamed I would be alive at this age, or have a wife and three daughters, yet neither did I dream I would suffer such pain or heartbreak. Still, there I was, seeing further down the road than ever before.

Sitting on those chancel steps, I felt guilty, almost sad. I had thought of those who'd been lost along the way, whether in body, spirit, or both. And, like so many times before, I wondered why I had survived.

My sadness was tempered by an extraordinary sense of gratefulness. We had stood, my family and I, as waters rose around us, and—by God's grace alone—we made something of life—the constant struggle, the unexpected joys, and the sense that each day does matter. Most of the hard stuff became part of the greater context of my life, not the other way around. Such perspective has been one of God's greatest gifts to me.

None of us, I reflected, knows how the journey will turn out. I had no idea that I would live this long or be privileged to be a part of so many wonderful adventures. For one reason or another—and I credit the hand of God—my body has held out longer than expected. I want my life to testify to something beyond my own survival. It is possible that I won't live to see this book published—possible even that I will die tomorrow. Though the odds may be different, this is no less true for you than for me, a reality that often leads to guilt and regret.

Are there choices I would prefer to do over again? Certainly. But framing our story within the context of God's love and grace reshapes our narrative and helps us see that, even in our mistakes, there is something bigger and better at work.

What must it have taken for three young Jewish exiles to choose to be thrown into a blazing furnace? How could Shadrach, Meshach, and Abednego have anticipated the fruit that their seemingly illogical, unreasonable act of faithfulness would bear?

When we choose the fire, we often find the meaning of our

lives. Each of us, each day, is close to the flames, and it is only natural that we think about running as fast as we can in the opposite direction.

This isn't just theological hindsight. Yes, I've emerged from the fire—from many fires—but like the three men in Daniel 3, I've emerged as a changed person. Nothing is the same after we step into the flames; nothing is easy.

Simple, perhaps, but never easy.

All God asks, I reflected as I sat on the steps of my empty church, *is that we do the thing he has given to us.* What comes next is up to him. All I can do is go home to my wife and daughters, laughing around our lunch table, and thank God for another day. In the morning, I can begin work on next week's sermon— and, as I do, thank God for yet another day.

The next several days after that first sermon in Gulf Breeze, I drove back and forth from our home in Mississippi to our new home in Florida, meeting movers on both ends and helping organize the transition. On one trip, I detoured to Pearl River County in South Mississippi and went by the family home where my grandparents lived.

Although no one in our family had lived there for many years, I stopped and knocked on the door. The young lady who came to the door was surprised, but after I explained who I was and that I wanted to walk through the backyard for a moment, she seemed less concerned. She had known my grandparents and said to take as much time as I wanted.

I walked through the backyard and even sat on the same bench where I had played as a child. So many dreams were born in that little garden. Dreaming was easier back then.

When I left the house, I drove a few miles down the road,

past our old church, and stopped at the field where my grandfather and I would sit under the peach trees. The trees were long gone, and new homes now cover most of the field, but there is one small section still available to walk in. As I stood in silence, I could have sworn that if I held my nose just right, I could still smell my grandfather's pipe tobacco and the faintest hint of peaches.

An hour later I found myself sitting on the hillside overlooking the golf course where my grandfather and I had played so many rounds and where, years earlier, I had sat with him and pondered what was "next." This patch of grass was, I realized, a holy place, for it was here that wisdom and prayers flowed from one generation to the next. It was here that Grandpa helped me see down the road just far enough to begin my own journey in the right direction.

On this day, I stood there thinking about *that* conversation, the one neither of us wanted to have but the one that changed my life forever. I thought about how far the road had taken me from that uncertain moment when a grandfather tried to comfort the grandson he thought he would soon lose to death.

Grandpa had walked through many flames in the course of his life, but now he gloried in the light of an everlasting sunrise, gifted to him by the risen Son. I, too, have walked through many flames, and many more will flare along my path, each one a chance to choose self-pity.

I pictured my grandfather, puffing his pipe sagaciously on this very patch of grass. *If anybody has a right to get in the corner and have a pity party about this, it's you. But as bad as this seems— and I know it's bad—you have a choice to make.*

The golf course stretched out below me like a green ocean.

I think you are going to make a choice other than pity, retreat, or surrender. I think you are going to live each day to the fullest with everything you have. I think you are going to take each day, no matter how many you have, and make something of it.

Grandpa knew me better than I knew myself. The more I see of life, and the more I see the guiding hand of God, the more convinced I am of Grandpa's wisdom. Each day we are given is a chance to live God's story—the wildest, most creative, most wonderful story ever told.

Each day I wake up to this choice.

No one, said Grandpa, *can ask any more of you.*

It is God's grace, and God's mercy, that he never asks any less.

NO ORDINARY FAIRY TALE

Pokey Stanford

Once in a while right in the middle of an ordinary life, love gives you a fairy tale. That just might best describe how I feel about this journey of life with Shane. He would be embarrassed by that characterization. I believe you have learned over these pages that Shane does not like the spotlight for himself. And if you did not catch that in him, I hope you will believe it when I say it to you. Shane's story, our story, has never been easy to tell. Shane has written lots of books that include snippets of the story, but ultimately he wants you, me, us to point back to God. It is that simple with him. Watching him agonize over telling the whole of his own story has both impressed and strained me because I knew how difficult it was for him and how much he would rather have just told you about the love of God and moved on.

But that is not what God called us to do. God wanted us to tell *this* story — all of it. Many friends who read parts of our journey they had not known before asked, "Why in the world would you share that?" Well, we debated, prayed, and struggled over what to share and what not to share for months. We would write a piece, scrap it, then include it, then scrap it again, only, by the end of the day, to see it back in the manuscript. At times it was a bit like being asked to strip bare in front of strangers. We felt vulnerable, fragile, and unsure.

Then God would step in again and dose us with his magnificent peace, and we would know that we had done the right thing. Of course, there are parts of the story I wish we had not told, but not because of what you think. I wish we didn't have to tell them is the reason. We walked so far away from God and from each other that sometimes I can still feel the grief of those moments. I hate the way our life turned out of control. But at the same time, I cannot express the joy of what we have found on the other side. We share so much because we have found so many in our ministry together who have been down similar paths and simply given up. We wanted to show people that life, regardless of how difficult and how much struggle, does not have to end the way the Adversary says it does. No, this pain, this guilt, this shame, this bad choice, this feeling of never being good enough—that is what is not normal in God's redemptive story. We are his sons and daughters, and that counts for something.

As I read our story again, I was not so much amazed at what we have been through as much as I was amazed at what God does so well and beautifully and completely in the midst of us. I remembered once again why I love my husband so much and why I consider our relationship such a blessing. Our marriage, our life together has been refined by fire. We have been through many tests and trials, and have found that through honest conversation and grace-filled prayer truly anything is possible. God is good through all of our turns and twists, trials and tribulation, joy and jubilation.

How have we endured the journey and not just survived, but prevailed? First, we have been blessed that God never took his eyes off of us. Even when we didn't feel it, we were loved unconditionally. Second, my husband is as amazing a man as you might imagine. Certainly he is a wonderful husband and father. But he is also a true friend and a remarkable child of God. He believes and lives what he preaches. I haven't witnessed this just in his walk and dealings with others. I have been privileged to watch him share that with me as well. What you have read and experienced in this book is genuine. Truly, Shane is as you read him.

The journey has not been fair to Shane in so many ways. What most don't see are the ways getting out of bed and going through another day are a struggle for him — the shots twice a day that are leaving his body sore and scarred, the increasing daily pain facing an aging hemophiliac, the fatigue after his heart surgery, and the handfuls of medicine that he takes daily just to stay with us. I'm certain along the journey that for him to want to go home would have been easier, but truly God is not finished with him yet (and I'm so glad)! Shane rarely complains and daily puts all of those he meets in front of his own needs. His living with chronic illness has not altered his outlook on life, but instead has given him insight into different facets along the way. I know I am prejudiced, but Shane is an amazing man of God!

People will often ask me if Shane and I have a "real marriage." I'm not always sure what that means, but most of the time they are referring to intimacy. The answer is a resounding yes. In that regard, as well as in every other aspect of our marriage, we have a very real marriage. But there is much more to our relationship. We are best friends and each other's biggest fans, and we genuinely appreciate and value the other's thoughts and considerations. We laugh, cry, and pray together and share intimate moments.

We also love being parents together. Our girls provide a focus and purpose that serve as an underserved blessing for us. Our life together is as real and as normal day-to-day as anyone's. And we fuss about the same things that others fuss about — money, the laundry, schedules, and keeping the house clean. Yes, our lives are very much like everyone else's, except that at the end of the day, we have a couple of other issues on our minds that never really go away. But it is the normal side of our life that makes the more unique, unusual parts of the path so special and meaningful. We've learned to live as life happens.

If I had to sum up what Shane's journey has meant to me, I would say that although we live daily with HIV and hep C, they do not dictate who we are. We have been together for longer than we have been apart. Sure, there are many days I wish I could get back for the both of us, but we must trust daily that God's grace, faithfulness, and forgiveness are sufficient to ease the pain along the way and to both offer and receive forgiveness for mistakes made. We have long moved on, because we caught a glimpse of what moving on could mean. And yes, it is even more wonderful than we had imagined. This season of our marriage has offered a great sense of renewal, and with everything that we have faced, I would not want to miss one single moment of what God has in store.

I hope Shane's words have offered you encouragement along your journey, and that you can see God's grace within them. Shane's heart for you is also one of the reasons I love him so. He has prayed for you and for what you would read from day one. He doesn't even know you, but he loves you.

And that is why I love him. We are so blessed because we realized what blessing really meant. And we learned to make life matter instead of just letting life go when it got too hard. No matter the dints, scrapes, bruises, or wounds, we are God's and we are together. And I would consider that a very *positive life*.

SPEECH AT THE GLOBAL AIDS SUMMIT, 2006

As a person living with HIV and AIDS, my entire life has been a race. A race against illness and disease, against fear and uncertainty, against discrimination and prejudice. A race against time.

Sure, the race has been difficult with many twists and turns — from growing up a hemophiliac to discovering my HIV status at sixteen to watching how the secrecy of my HIV status affected the emotional life of our family and relationships.

It is a journey with spiritual struggles and tension — from watching my denomination's struggle over whether to ordain me to being rejected by the first church to which I was appointed as pastor.

And certainly, it is a race with great loss and disillusionment — from the loss of dear friends to the disease to the loss of others for the fear surrounding it.

No, it has not been easy, pushing me to trust beyond what I can see and understand, even, at times, pressing the limits of my faith, not necessarily as much for God as for God's people.

Certainly this is not a path that I would have chosen. But

oddly enough, so many miles into it now, I would also not trade it with anyone.

You see, HIV has also afforded me an incredible glimpse into the best of what God offers in this world and the best for what God's people can become. This journey informs me, in God's call for each of us, to respond faithfully as God's children, and teaches all of us who call ourselves "Christian" important lessons that potentially can change our world.

Lessons about time. Because of my illness, I am reminded each day that time is a privilege given to us by God, a luxury afforded to us with the possibility that each of us can make a difference in this world.

Lessons about relationships. I am blessed with a beautiful wife, three wonderful daughters, and countless family members and friends who remind me that the most important things we do in this world are not done alone.

Lessons about simplicity. More, bigger, and *nicer* pale in comparison to simple things like sunsets with those you love and the laughter of children at play.

And most important, *lessons about real faith.* Personally, HIV reminds me every day that, with God's grace, what I need I have, and what I have is sufficient. Sufficient to confront the struggles of my health and the uncertainties of tomorrow. Sufficient to meet the needs of others if we, the body of Christ, might agree to meet them together. For still, more than anything I have ever known, the body of Christ (when we truly live like it), with all of its imperfections, holds as the hope of the world, bearing witness to this amazing gospel that says God passionately loves the unlovable, the marginalized, and the forgotten.

No, HIV is not easy for any of us. But it is a journey with

real lessons for real life, and if we listen carefully, it can teach us much about loving God and each other.

Friends, we have a race to run. This world cannot afford to run it alone.

NINE LESSONS FROM A POSITIVE LIFE

A Study and Reflection Guide

Over the past months, I have roamed through mountains of journal entries, listened to stories from family members and friends, sat quietly while I made notes from old memories of events long passed, and prayed that God would open my mind and my heart in order to tell the most honest, most faithful recollection of my life's journey possible. I have written a lot before this project—books, articles, poetry even—but nothing like this.

Many times in writing this book my focus gravitated away from my story and from my message. I realized in so many places that the story doesn't belong just to me, but also to the countless family and friends whose lives crossed my path. The story certainly belongs to my mom, too, who as a twenty-two-year-old mother, remembered one day, long forgotten, that her father had been a "free bleeder." The story also belongs to my grandfather, who watched as his grandson navigated deep issues of life and death at a time when most teenagers would have worried about girls and sports and other teenage things. The story belongs to my doctor and, later, friend, Ronnie Kent, who wrestled for years with the fact that he had been the one who had prescribed the Factor that was contaminated with the HIV that had run through my blood system. It would be years before he would verbalize that great burden and discuss the weight it had laid on his life. Certainly, the story belongs to Pokey, the fifteen-year-old girl who sat in the boy's lap on the school trip not knowing that her life would never be the same again. Her own illnesses and baggage were tied so heavily to her that they were as wounding and damaging as any physical disease could be. And of course, the story belongs to my children, to my friends, to my parishioners, and even to those who do not know me but have heard some sermon or seen some article that has told, through my circumstances, of how God loves us in spite of traumatic prognoses. This story also belongs to you, for I believe that God's commission to share my story with you is why I have survived this long.

I am just one character in this drama, moving from one act to another. The real protagonist is a Jewish carpenter who taught us that even the most mundane of our days means something wrapped within his grace, and that the sweetest ways by which we will experience them will be done with others who love him too. Each day is filled with lessons that we *should* learn. God places them there, around our tables, at the edge of our hospital beds, in the air of strained relationships and conversations, on the cusp of our new beginnings, that we might see the deeper place and purpose of life.

Several years ago I was asked to write an article listing the lessons I have learned from my journey with HIV/AIDS. The result was a list of nine lessons that measure my story and my journey. They include life questions I asked along the way, Scriptures that came to define my connection to God, and challenges to how I see God and his work in the world. They sum up in a few words, along with their Scripture references, why I feel so blessed and so insistent on making my story more than just about me. Over the next few pages, I list them for you. I believe you will see the same indications of God's grace and presence as you work through them. And I believe God will show you something beautiful about the positive life he has in store for you too.

Just as you have worked your way through this story, contemplating your own story of how God has walked with you and has called you to see your path differently and better, I encourage you to look at these lessons as another conversation starter, one that creates in you your own list of qualities and principles that God has been teaching you. Reflect on them, and maybe, just maybe, you will see another angle or opportunity where God is working or can work in you.

These lessons are part Bible study, part reflective guide, part catharsis. But mainly they are nuggets of how the story you just read taught me something that I share, not because I want your story to look like mine, but because our story should look like God's. Maybe, as you have read the book and seen parts of yourself or even new parts of God's grace that you had forgotten was present in all of us, you have wanted to ask other questions, to go deeper into the lessons. Here is your chance.

I invite you to grab your Bible, your journal, your pencil or pen, and spend a few extra moments with me.

LESSON 1: BECOME SATISFIED WITH NEVER BEING SATISFIED.

Overview: Life is about moving forward. We either follow or lead. Deciding which we will do makes all the difference. But many of us, especially when confronted with difficult life issues, end up settling for less than life's best opportunities. God wants more for us and from us. He wants us to be at peace with life but not be complacent toward living out and sharing his grace.

Questions: In what ways have you grown complacent in your spiritual walk? Have the troubles of life defined your view of the possibilities of life? How does learning to make the best of our circumstances reframe our potential for making a difference in our world?

Scripture: 1 Corinthians 15:58

Consider: Three principles for defining life before it has a chance to define you.

1. Develop a strong connection to your devotional life through a consistent study of God's Word.
2. Make a "joy journal" in which you name your joys. I have kept one for years, and it is helpful, especially when life is difficult, to look back on the joys I have named. As the old hymn says, "Count your blessings; name them one by one."
3. Continue to work and serve. Everything you do for God has a purpose and is useful for his work in the world.

LESSON 2: CRAVE AWE AND WONDER.

Overview: Have you ever watched a child on Christmas morning? God shapes life to experience the wonder of his creation. Every day is a gift and should be opened as such. The first-century Christians, even with all of their struggles and obstacles, experienced awe and wonder because they saw the working of God in the midst of their daily routines. Finding God in the small, simple things is the most profound opportunity for seeing God in our daily routines. Remember, God is in the whispers.

Questions: Describe the areas of "awe and wonder" in your life. What brings you joy? What keeps you from celebrating what God is doing in your life? How do the simple "wonders" of God's day impact our journey? What keeps us from seeing how God is working around us?

Scripture: 1 Kings 19:12

Consider: Four ways not to miss the awe and wonder of God around and in your life.

1. Make a "little things" list of small kindnesses that people do for you.
2. Reciprocate by paying kindness forward. Share a small kindness with someone else but dedicate it to a friend.
3. A letter a day; recover the art of writing a letter or, if you must, an email to encourage a friend.
4. Instead of just a prayer list, also establish a blessings list at your church or through a small group or by yourself. Find a way to share it with others.

LESSON 3: SIMPLIFY.

Overview: We complicate life, not the other way around. As life grows more complicated, we have one of two basic reactions: we either recoil from it or jump into the storm. Neither is healthy. We must learn to meet life as we find it and then prioritize according to what God would have us do in our lives. Most of our priorities are driven by our ambitions, not by God's plan for our lives.

Questions: Write down the ten most important things you want to accomplish. Then tear the list in half. What keeps your life so complicated and charged? Is it relationships? Priorities? Duties? Expectations? Some of each? How can you enrich life by simplifying your priorities and redefining your goals and values? What do the Beatitudes from Jesus' Sermon on the Mount teach us about ordering our lives into manageable frames for living?

Scripture: Matthew 5:1 – 12

Consider: Three principles Christ teaches in the Sermon on the Mount about the ordering of life.

1. "He sat down. . . ." Jesus focused on the important concepts first.
2. "He opened his mouth. . . ." Jesus made transparency a way of life. To live openly and honestly is a first step to living simply.
3. "He taught them saying. . . ." Jesus did the important things over and over again. He repeated the critical steps and added value to them instead of trying to do too many things at one time.

LESSON 4: CELEBRATE BOLDLY AND LAUGH LOUDLY.

Overview: In Luke 15, God seeks after lost things and then throws a party when they are found. Put simply, Christians don't throw parties and laugh enough. There is much to be down about in our world, but nothing recharges our instincts, intentions, and desires for living like Christ than joy and sharing that joy with others.

Questions: After reading Luke 15, which character are you most like? Are you the younger brother, breaking the rules and allowing your joy to be stolen? Are you the older brother, making rules your religion and allowing your joy to be stolen? Or are you the Father, who with reckless love and grace, sees the joy of life even with its struggles? Deciding which character we are determines how we experience consistent, bold joy in this world.

Scripture: Read Luke 15 and the stories of the lost sheep, lost coin, and lost son.

Consider: Three principles about God, joy, and lost things.

1. God loves lost things — that is, he has extravagant, ridiculous love for the most broken parts of our lives.
2. God is always watching for the horizon to see if we will return to him. Nothing, by far, brings him more joy than this.
3. God celebrates when a lost or broken life is brought home or back together. Why don't we?

LESSON 5: DO LIFE WITH OTHERS.

Overview: The most important things we do in this world can't be done alone. The Bible is full of one story after another of God building community. Whether it is the garden of Eden, Jacob's children, David's broken family, the disciples, or the early church, God loves for humanity to experience life in the same fullness and interdependence that God experiences the Trinity — Father, Son, and Holy Spirit. Of course, it doesn't always happen, and the results are more than obvious. What about your journey? Do you live life as a lone ranger, or are you involved with people? The difference is great.

Questions: Make a list of the most important relationships in your life. Do they offer a positive source of encouragement, or do they drain life? Why? Why is "doing life" with others so difficult? What are the benefits of sharing the journey with others? How can being in community and being vulnerable in your faith journey provide a sense of depth, stability, and safety for you? What is required of *you* in doing life together with others?

Scripture: Acts 2:42–47

Consider: Four devotions of the first Christians in their life together.

1. *Teaching and learning.* One of the best and most beneficial ways to do life together is by learning the Word of God together.
2. *Fellowship.* Sharing a meal, laughing, and crying together are all part of God's greater plan that we might experience life with others.
3. *Sacraments.* Sharing in the holy sacraments together allows us to experience the sacred places of God together. Sharing "real moments" and service with brothers and sisters in Christ changes the dynamics of relationships and makes them significant.
4. *Prayer and devotion.* Investing oneself with others in a devotional life and regimen of prayer focuses the group on the greater good and shifts the group's dynamics from being a support/gripe/gossip/whine group to a group committed to making a difference in each other's lives.

LESSON 6: EMBRACE THE UNFAMILIAR.

Overview: The measure of persons is found not in what they know, but in what they are willing to admit they don't know.

This is also true for what we are unsure of and afraid of for the future. God's plan, as I have learned in my life, is not always clear on the front end. But it is amazingly clear as we look back and see his hand. Part of the process of living out God's work in our lives is the journey itself and learning to trust him along the way.

Questions: Reading Romans 8, we get a glimpse into Paul's own questions for God. This work is more treatise than letter. What are Paul's concerns about the journey? Can you sense his own uncertainties at points? Paul makes a dramatic shift in the middle of the passage for the reader. What is it? How does Paul see the future for a believer, even in the midst of difficult times? What does it mean for Paul to say that nothing will separate us from Christ?

Scripture: Romans 8

Consider: Three aspects of Paul's view of God's unfailing love and guidance.

1. Paul draws a distinct line between the difficulties of the world and the hope we find in Christ.
2. Paul's litany of "troubles" includes spiritual, emotional, and physical threats.
3. It is the love of God that is the momentum of Christ's life, work, and salvation in and for us.

LESSON 7: LOVE UNCONDITIONALLY.

Overview: This lesson should speak for itself. None of us are perfect. All of us have those broken places, which when they are revealed to the light, look ugly and unlovable. On our own, we cannot experience the kind of acceptance and wholeness that

God desires. However, agape changes the rules. It is unconditional love practiced by the Creator for a broken creation. It runs counterintuitively to the consensus of how we often order the world: "I will love you based on how you love me." But that is not the way God has ordered the redemptive process in his economy. The sooner we come to grips with what this means for each of us, for our lives and also for how we treat each other, the better we will see the Creator.

Questions: What does it mean to love unconditionally? What about those who continue to do things that are harmful or abusive? How does God make provisions for loving the sinner but hating the sin? In more common settings and situations, how does unconditional love enrich our relationships and change the way we communicate and redefine our priorities? How does the unconditional love of God through Christ model how we are to love one another?

Scripture: John 3:16 and 1 John 4:7 – 8

Consider: Five principles for understanding the unconditional love of God.

1. *Parameters.* God's love knows no parameters. As much as God hates the brokenness of our lives, he loves us even more.
2. *Personal.* God's love for us is personal and individual. He doesn't sit back unconnected from our struggles and situations.
3. *Provision.* God's loves makes provision for our brokenness and for our own inability to rectify the hurts and haunted corners of our soul.
4. *Proximity.* God's love draws us closer to him by him becoming like us in Christ.

5. *Powerful.* God's love is powerful and complete, and what he offers in Christ is eternal.

LESSON 8: GET YOUR HANDS AND FEET DIRTY.

Overview: Holy is not about cleanliness; it is about proximity. Jesus loved "the least of these"; so should we. This lesson means more to me that any of the others. I thought surviving my own struggle was enough. It wasn't. God meant for me to respond to the needs of my brothers and sisters as though my own body were perfect. There is always someone with a more complicated situation, sadder story, or more broken path. The only way to move forward is to pry away the broken nature of our sin that separates us from God and land in the middle of the world's problems with love, grace, and solutions.

Questions: How does helping our brothers and sisters in need draw us closer to God? What is it about Matthew 25 that stunned those listening? How does helping others help us to see Jesus clearer? In Mark 1 the leper makes a bold statement. What is it? How does the "willingness" of Jesus trump the other attributes or points of the interaction? Why does that question redefine how faith and love intersect in our own lives?

Scripture: Matthew 25; Mark 1:40–45

Consider: Three points from the story of the man with leprosy.

1. We have people in need all around us. The man had sat at the gate for a long time, begging from many people.
2. Often the issue is not ability but willingness to make a difference. The man asked Jesus a different kind of question. The key was his willingness.

3. Once you are touched by God, something happens and you can't hold it in. The man could not contain his joy and excitement.

LESSON 9: READ MORE FAIRY TALES AND RIDE MORE ROLLER COASTERS.

Overview: Fairy tales and roller coasters are like life: between "Once upon a time" and "happily ever after," there are turns, twists, and ups and downs; but in the end, it is worth the adventure. Life is an adventure, and we need to learn to navigate the adventure or it can overwhelm us. Most of what we miss in terms of really important moments of our lives has little to do with scheduled activities or marks on a to-do list. The critical elements of life's most personal and poignant places happen when we take down the shades and take a look at what's behind the curtains.

Questions: What keeps us from enjoying the "real moments" of life? Is your life more about control or about experiencing the joy of what God can do in and through you? God adds color to our day and to our journey when we stop to take a deep breath and soak up the experience of life. We serve a God who is always doing something new, something wonderful, beautiful, and exciting. We must be careful not to thwart the adventures he has for us by overmanaging our lives.

Scripture: Psalm 149

Consider: Three requirements for the new song God sings in us.

1. *Always sing.* We are born to sing a song of hope and joy.
2. *Always praise.* The focus of our lives is not to be our agendas, to-do lists, or need to make another buck. The focus is God.

3. *Always rejoice.* At the end of the day, the work of God is greater in us than what the world teaches us to value. We are his; thus we are bound by his grace and potential in us. The length and width and depth of our lives are not measured by the standards of this world. The adventure belongs to God. And we belong to him.

ACKNOWLEDGMENTS

Life is more than the sum of what we can say. I started this project with these words, and they are no less true as I finish. With as much as I have written within these pages, no book could hold everything I would want to say to those who have meant so much to me along the journey. Thus, to everyone who has guided me with thoughts and prayers, I offer a heartfelt thank-you. Your name may not be listed here, but I hope you know who you are and how much you mean to me.

The following is my feeble attempt to list individuals who remain at the center of just about everything I am and all that I do. They are the cheering squad, yes, but also my balance when life gets out of control. If it weren't for these people, none of this story would be possible.

To my editor, Angela Scheff, and everyone at Zondervan, for making this process much easier than it should have been.

To Chip MacGregor, a wonderful agent and friend, for being convinced that what I have to say truly means something.

To dear friends and marvelous people whom I dreamed of meeting—Kay, Rick, Deanna, and Paulette. When I finally did, I was astounded that we, in the sweetest and simplest forms, became friends. Thank you for remarkable lives and testimonies that inform and challenge me every day.

To my friends and colleagues in ministry, especially our family at Gulf Breeze UMC, for your support and patience.

To our community groups and countless friends who keep us grounded and faithful through very busy lives to always "do life together" — Ronnie and Anne, Robert and Jill, Dawson and Brenda, Gloria and Joey, Don and Lawrie, Bill and Beth, Bo and Leigh Anne, and Darryl.

To my pals and partners in crime, Anthony and Bo, thanks for the attitude adjustments and the unwavering faith.

To the countless medical professionals who cared for me over the years, and who, over the course of the journey, also became dear friends. Nancy, Mike, Nagen, Joe, Chuck, Rathi, Betty, and Connie, words are inadequate.

To my family, Mom, Buford, Whitney, Dad, Patty, Nanny, Delana, Tracy, Randy, Kimberly, and Memaw for, once more, believing in me more than I believe in myself.

To Sarai Grace, Juli Anna, and Emma Leigh, for being my sweet reasons to make the most of every moment. I love you.

To Pokey, for the journey, through good and bad, I wouldn't trade one single moment. You are my treasure. I love you.

And to Jesus, my dearest Friend, for making more of me than I was able and for sharing more with me than I deserve.

FOR FURTHER READING

Bell, James Stuart, with Anthony Palmer Dawson. *From the Library of C. S. Lewis: Selections from Writers Who Influenced His Spiritual Journey*. Colorado Springs: Shaw, 2004.

Bonhoeffer, Dietrich. *Letters and Papers from Prison*. New York: Macmillan, 1953.

Bunyan, John. *The Pilgrim's Progress*. London: Penguin, 1965.

McKinley, Rick. *Jesus in the Margins*. Sisters, Ore.: Multnomah, 2005.

Miller, Donald. *To Own a Dragon*. Colorado Springs: NavPress, 2006.

Saltzman, David. *The Jester Has Lost His Jingle*. Palos Verdes Estates, Calif.: Jester, 1995.

See, Carolyn. *Making a Literary Life*. New York: Ballantine, 2002.

Sjogren, Steve, and Rob Lewin. *Community of Kindness*. Rev. ed. Ventura, Calif.: Regal, 2003.

Stanford, Shane. *When God Disappears*. Ventura, Calif.: Regal, 2008.

Verghese, Abraham. *The Tennis Partner*. New York: HarperCollins, 1998.

Share Your Thoughts

With the Author: Your comments will be forwarded to the author when you send them to *zauthor@zondervan.com*.

With Zondervan: Submit your review of this book by writing to *zreview@zondervan.com*.

Free Online Resources at

www.zondervan.com

Zondervan AuthorTracker: Be notified whenever your favorite authors publish new books, go on tour, or post an update about what's happening in their lives at www.zondervan.com/authortracker.

Daily Bible Verses and Devotions: Enrich your life with daily Bible verses or devotions that help you start every morning focused on God. Visit www.zondervan.com/newsletters.

Free Email Publications: Sign up for newsletters on Christian living, academic resources, church ministry, fiction, children's resources, and more. Visit www.zondervan.com/newsletters.

Zondervan Bible Search: Find and compare Bible passages in a variety of translations at www.zondervanbiblesearch.com.

Other Benefits: Register yourself to receive online benefits like coupons and special offers, or to participate in research.

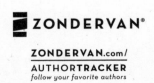

ZONDERVAN®

ZONDERVAN.com/
AUTHORTRACKER
follow your favorite authors